# WINNING
### *Tennis Nutrition*

# WINNING
## *Tennis Nutrition*

GRACE LEE, MS, RDN

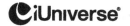

# WINNING TENNIS NUTRITION

iUniverse books may be ordered through booksellers or by contacting:

iUniverse
1663 Liberty Drive
Bloomington, IN 47403
www.iuniverse.com
1-800-Authors (1-800-288-4677)

ISBN: 978-1-4917-7329-1 (sc)
ISBN: 978-1-4917-7328-4 (e)

Library of Congress Control Number: 2015917715

Print information available on the last page.

iUniverse rev. date: 1/29/2016

# CONTENTS

# INTRODUCTION

If I told you that you could hit crisper volleys and brutal backhands by improving your diet, would you listen? Would you be willing to lose five or ten pounds to get to your next rating level? Would you pack the right snacks in your tennis bag to fuel your way through a three-hour singles match victory? Would you plan and time what you eat and drink in an all-day tournament to better your chances of adding a trophy to your boasting rights?

I know you would. Tennis players are driven athletes. No other sports venue involves one athlete competing head-to-head against the lone opposition across that distant net, battling in unpredictable weather conditions for an indefinite, seemingly infinite, amount of time. There are no innings, periods, or rounds. There is no coach or teammate (in singles tennis) by one's side. One missed or made shot could determine the match win or loss. Tennis has tremendous mental demand from start to finish, throughout the ebb and flow of ad ins and ad outs. Tennis is sport in a class by itself, making tennis players a unique breed of driven athlete seeking ways to play better and win.

With that said, a win or loss rests entirely on your shoulders. As an avid tennis player and a registered dietitian (RD) with an advanced degree in human nutrition from Cornell University—one of the world's top nutrition programs—I see tennis players at all levels search for the tennis holy grail. From intense drilling, weekly lessons, tennis camps, sports psychology, and fitness and conditioning, the one deficit I see in competitive club tennis—and even at the elite high school, collegiate, and professional levels—is the focus on nutrition specifically targeted at tennis performance.

Tennis sports nutrition must be in every player's "bag check" of training regimen and competitive play. There are no ifs, ands, or buts about this.

Sports nutrition is a specialized field that integrates nutrition with physical activity and athletic performance. Sports nutrition teaches athletes how to use food and fluids to train more effectively, stay healthy, and improve performance to gain that winning edge. With twenty-five years of experience working with clients and leading nutrition programs, I have seen many tennis players underestimate the value of sports nutrition.

Registered dietitians are nutrition professionals. RDs can be board certified in sports nutrition, holding the title of sports specialist in dietetics, or CSSD. RDs who are CSSDs have a minimum of two years of experience in sports nutrition, maintain 1,500 practice hours each year, and recertify by passing a challenging exam. If a CSSD is hard to come by in your tennis community, seek sound professional advice from an RD.

*Winning Tennis Nutrition* will teach you how to apply good tennis nutrition in practice. It will make a striking difference in your athletic performance. You will find this irrefutable after incorporating good nutrition into both your tennis training program and your competitive play. Proper nutrition and hydration on and off the court can mean the difference between a match win and loss. I have provided many tennis friends and acquaintances with nutritional advice. They are living proof that improved nutrition results in better fitness and greater confidence—which translates into winning tennis.

I recently interviewed American tennis prodigy Jimmy Arias, former number-five world-ranked tennis player in 1980 behind only the likes of tennis legends Jimmy Connors, John McEnroe, Ivan Lendl, and Mats Wilander. In 1979, at fifteen years of age,

Arias was the youngest player ever to reach a world ranking. He is now a popular commentator for ESPN and the Tennis Channel. Arias feels that nutrition, more than ever, is vital to today's tennis—now a much more physical, harder-hitting game than in his professional days. He agrees that the player who can run faster and last longer will invariably be the winner.[1] Nutrition plays a key role in optimizing the fitness level to do so.

I also interviewed Nick Bollettieri, world-renowned tennis coach and 2014 inductee to the International Tennis Hall of Fame. He is Founder and President Emeritus of the Bollettieri Tennis Program at IMG Academy in Bradenton, Florida. IMG Academy is the training mecca for the world's best athletes, tennis players included. Bollettieri is credited with developing tennis greats who need no first-name introduction: Sharapova, Agassi, Courier, Seles, and the Williams sisters—to name only a few. Like Arias, Bollettieri agrees that fitness and nutrition have never been more critical in a game that has evolved into such a physically demanding sport.[2]

Spanning a tennis and coaching career lasting six decades, this icon believes that nutrition is an integral part of physical conditioning, which needs to be individualized for each player. IMG Academy supports the role of nutrition in athletic performance, sporting both an on-site nutrition program and the Gatorade Sports Science Institute (GSSI), which is utilized by world-class athletes.

Beyond tennis, Bollettieri feels nutrition is far more important to overall mental and physical well-being. He adds, "If you don't eat right, you will falter, not only in tennis but in life—in all you do: in school and academia, in work, in simple tasks from picking up the house to mowing the lawn."[3] Good nutrition is key to success in life.

Tennis phenoms also agree. Their on-court tennis performance proves it. Realizing he had a gluten sensitivity, Novak Djokovic changed his diet, lost weight, improved his health, and underwent a rigorous physical conditioning program. The results: an astounding, incredulous 37–0 win streak, ten singles titles, and three of the four coveted Grand Slam trophies in 2011—a superb return on investment.

Andy Murray went from Grand Slam bridesmaid to 2012 US Open champion through physical conditioning, diet included. Murray's well-publicized diet program is a testament to how nutrition helped transform him into 2012 US Open winner. Murray won his most prestigious Grand Slam trophy, Wimbledon 2013, against none other than his superfit rival, Novak Djokovic.

Chapter 1 discusses nutritional guidelines in great detail. A solid foundation of good nutrition determines the efficacy of sports nutrition on tennis performance. Chapter 1 translates these nutritional guidelines into practice, offering tips for around-the-clock, high-performance eating.

In their quest to find the magic bullet to transform their game, tennis players, like many athletes, are drawn to supplements and ergogenic aids. Sifting through truth versus hype, chapter 2 discerns which supplements work and which do not. Chapter 2 also delivers tips for being a savvy supplements shopper.

Chapters 3, 4, and 5 discuss protein, fat, and carbohydrates. The proper proportion of protein, carbohydrates, and fat are essential not only for maintaining good nutrition but in enhancing sports performance. Sports nutrition and training regimens need to be adapted to each type of sport. *Winning Tennis Nutrition* provides practical advice on getting the right type and amount of carbohydrates, protein, and fat in the proper balance for optimal health and tennis performance.

Because the fitter the athlete, the better the athlete, addressing weight management is an essential discussion in tennis sports nutrition for all players: club, junior, collegiate, and professional levels. In 2010, American tennis star Mardy Fish dropped thirty pounds in three weeks on an unconventional diet plan. His weight loss and improved fitness level helped catapult him to a 2011 career-high ranking of number seven in the world—the highest-ranked American male player that year. This veteran player had this breakthrough year well into his tennis career.

Chapter 6 emphasizes the difference between weight loss and weight management—when dissected, two very different terms. Managing weight is a lifelong goal, while weight loss is all too frequently the transient action of losing weight. Chapter 6 offers insights and tips for successful weight management.

With most tennis played outdoors, where the tennis climate and court can be blistery hot, fluids before, during, and after play are vital to health and performance. Chapter 7 discusses the critically important role of fluids, including the amount and types necessary for peak tennis performance. This chapter analyzes many popular drink choices, from coconut water to energy drinks, as well as their place on and off the tennis court.

No tennis bag should leave home without a healthy snack. Fuel and fluids during a tennis match are just as important as what we eat before and afterward. Chapter 8 identifies the best snacks to pack in your tennis bag during a match—when on-court performance matters the most.

Many children in tennis academies dream of being the next international superstar. Children have different challenges with diet and nutrition compared to adults. Parents and coaches cannot ignore the integral role of good nutrition in both a child's training program and the pathway to healthy growth and development. Chapter 9 reviews nutritional needs of children in tennis along with the challenges they face in establishing good dietary habits. Practical tips for child, coach, and parent can help overcome the obstacles to good nutrition.

Chapter 10 organizes nutritional information into winning eating plans for various tennis match scenarios. Research clearly shows the benefits of nutrient timing—how we time foods and fluids for optimal tennis performance and recovery. Competing all day or over several days in a singles tournament requires game-day eating plans that time their nutrient delivery for peak performance.

In the final chapter, I conclude with a nutrition and fitness tribute to eighty-six-year-old Doris Jane Lutz. This tennis dynamo is currently the 2015 International Tennis Foundation's (ITF) number-one ladies player in the world in the eighty-five-year-old age group for women's singles. Through her words of wisdom, Lutz exemplifies how nutrition, fitness, and mental toughness have made her an international tennis champion at the ripe age of eighty-six.[4]

Each chapter presents an inspiring quote from the greatest tennis players of our time. These inspirational quotes are taken from Margaret Miller's *Enduring Words for the Athlete*. Each chapter also begins with real-life tennis nutrition case studies. Tennis players who have asked me for tips graciously share their stories on how diet has helped (or hindered) their tennis game.

A winning tennis player will succeed with certain tangible and intangible qualities. These include an undying will to succeed, coupled with the determination to do so; meeting personal goals—health, fitness, and nutrition included; and the unremitting perseverance through hard work (the blood, sweat, and tears) that makes tennis the enticing sport we love to play.

# 1

# GOOD NUTRITION EQUALS GREAT TENNIS

**Champions keep playing until they get it right.**
—Billie Jean King

Alan, an avid and competitive club player rated at the 4.5 USTA level, came up to me at our tennis club, declaring we "need to straighten out my diet." He was trying to lose weight to improve his on-court fitness level. When I asked how, he responded matter-of-factly, "A low-carb, high-protein diet." Knowing Alan plays at least three times a week in the hot Florida climate, I asked him how he felt during his matches. He responded, "Lousy," having reduced stamina and energy to carry a singles match from start to finish with the same mojo. Alan was excluding food groups—primarily carbohydrates—along with their essential vitamins, minerals, phytonutrients, and fiber in a diet lacking variety. The culprit: inadequate nutrition. Great tennis requires great nutrition.

# EATING TO STAY HEALTHY

Just like solid ground strokes and superb footwork are the foundation of tennis, good nutrition is essential to overall health and wellness. Proper nutrition enhances the efficacy of tennis sports nutrition. Any sports nutrition regimen will flounder if proper nutrition is not at its base. Many tennis players resort to a variety of diets and supplements before they even examine whether or not their eating plan is nutritionally sound.

Leading health organizations promote evidence-based dietary guidelines for diet and nutrition. A few of these organizations include the American Heart Association (AHA), the American College of Sports Medicine (ACSM), Institute of Medicine (IOM), National Cancer Institute (NCI), and the Academy of Nutrition and Dietetics (AND). *Evidence-based* means that research supports or substantiates nutritional findings. Evidence distinguishes nutrition fact from nutrition hype.

Nutrition is a complex science, requiring evidence to support diet and nutrition claims. Indeed, hearing the latest nutrition news from television, Internet sites, and social media (to name a few) can cause conflicting information overload. A mixed blessing in being readily accessible, this information can be unproven, unreplicated, or frankly erroneous, often based on hype and personal anecdotes—not evidence.

Why are consumers lured by the appeal of the latest nutrition buzz or diet trend, forsaking more sound nutritional principles based on evidence? In part, they are culpable of relying on the media for nutritional advice. Today's media is not solely television and newspaper. Information is gathered from blogs and chat rooms; web-based searches; vitamin and supplement shops; countless beauty, nutrition, and fitness magazines; and even unlicensed practitioners who may provide unsound, often unsafe, nutritional advice. This information can be completely unfounded. Like wildfire, the information spreads when shared by the likes of tweets, Facebook, blogs, and other social media. The information is literally at our fingertips and frequently oversimplified, hence easily misinterpreted.

Sports nutrition is a contemporary science. Consumers want to stay up to date. Like fashion, the latest diet trends can be much more exciting than practical information derived from scientific evidence and critical thinking. Packaged and marketed the right way, this information can be instantly sold to even the most astute consumer.

The field of nutrition is in its golden age. Today, researchers focus on how components in the variety of foods we eat promote health and wellness and improve athletic performance, whereas only a few decades ago, professionals focused on nutrition's role in preventing deficiency diseases. It truly is an exciting time for this emerging and dynamic field. New developments unfold on a daily basis. This is the nature of nutritional science—it is never stagnant.

Finally, there may be an institutionalized cynicism toward scientific experts who use evidence to make public health policy. This scrutiny can make consumers skeptical of policy and more trusting of independent sources, which may or may not have credibility. When people resort to unsubstantiated nutritional advice, they may be doing more harm to their health than good. Analyzing nutritional information from all sources is beneficial. Seek the assistance of professionals, such as a registered dietitian (RD), to help put evidence-based nutritional information into practice.

The public policy standard for nutritional guidelines for Americans is set by the US Department of Agriculture (USDA) and the Department of Health and Human Services (DHHS). Every five years, the USDA and the DHHS revise the Dietary Guidelines for Americans based on current, updated evidence. The newest revision will produce the forthcoming 2015 dietary guidelines.

These recommendations for Americans two years of age and older focus on eating a diet to promote health, prevent disease, and maintain a healthy weight. These guidelines are familiar to many of us. However, very few of us incorporate them as our foundation for nutrition and fitness.

The 2010 dietary guidelines are listed below.[5] Keep in mind that these are general guidelines, a broad framework, from which you build your tennis nutrition plan. Sports nutrition goes well beyond these dietary guidelines. As you patiently read through them, think about whether your diet meets these targets.*

## 2010 US DIETARY GUIDELINES FOR AMERICANS (USDA/DHHS)

### BALANCING CALORIES TO MANAGE WEIGHT

- Prevent and/or reduce obesity through improved eating and physical activity behaviors.
- Control total caloric intake. For people who are overweight or obese, this means consuming fewer calories from both food and beverages.
- Increase physical activity, while decreasing time spent in sedentary behaviors.
- Maintain appropriate caloric balance at each life stage: childhood, adolescence, pregnancy and breastfeeding, and older age.

### FOODS AND FOOD COMPONENTS TO REDUCE

- Reduce daily sodium intake to fewer than 2,300 milligrams. Americans fifty-one years of age or older should reduce sodium intake to 1,500 milligrams or fewer as well as people of any age who are African American or have hypertension, diabetes, or chronic kidney disease. The 1,500 milligrams sodium intake applies to about 50 percent of Americans.
- Consume less than 10 percent of calories from saturated fats, replacing them with monounsaturated or polyunsaturated sources.

---

*The 2015 revised Dietary Guidelines were issued in January, 2016.

- Consume fewer than 300 milligrams per day of dietary cholesterol.
- Keep trans-fatty acid consumption as low as possible.
- Reduce the intake of calories from solid fats and sugars.
- Limit the consumption of foods that contain refined grains.
- If alcohol is consumed, it should be consumed in moderation—up to one drink per day for women and two drinks per day for men.

## FOOD AND NUTRIENTS TO INCREASE

- Increase vegetable and fruit intake.
- Eat a variety of vegetables, especially dark-green, red, and orange vegetables, as well as beans and peas.
- Consume at least half of all grains as whole grains. Replace refined grains with whole grains.
- Increase intake of fat-free or low-fat milk and dairy products, such as yogurt, cheese, or fortified soy beverages.
- Increase the amount and variety of seafood by choosing seafood in place of fatty cuts of meat or poultry.
- Replace protein foods that are higher in solid fats with choices that are lower in solid fats, calories, and/or sources of oils.
- Use oils to replace solid fats where possible.
- Choose foods that provide more potassium, dietary fiber, calcium, and vitamin D, which are nutrients of concern in American diets. These foods include vegetables, fruits, whole grains, and milk and milk products.

## BUILDING HEALTHY EATING PATTERNS

- Select an eating pattern that meets nutrient needs over time at an appropriate calorie level.
- Account for all foods and beverages consumed and assess how they fit within a total healthy eating pattern.
- Follow food safety recommendations when preparing and eating foods to reduce the risk of food-borne illness.

One seemingly enigmatic message that has not been the central focus of dietary policy guidelines until recently is portion control. Most tennis players can identify foods that are more nutritious than others. Even a nutrition novice realizes an orange is a healthier tennis snack option than a doughnut.

But finding the proper balance of foods in the proper portion sizes has eluded Americans. The fact that almost two-thirds of adults and one-third of children in the United States are overweight, defined as being 10 percent or more above ideal body weight, supports the challenge in overcoming portion distortion. More than one-third of Americans are obese, defined as being 20 percent or more above ideal body weight.[6]

The prevalence of people who are overweight or obese is a serious public health concern—an understatement. Being overweight or obese are risk factors for many chronic diseases, such as hypertension, diabetes, stroke, cancer, and heart disease. Obesity aggravates degenerative joint disease, such as osteoarthritis—joint conditions that tennis players may experience in their life spans. Some experts identify obesity as a symptom of the true culprits hurting America's health: poor diet and lack of activity.

These diseases cause morbidity (illness) and mortality (death) in many Americans. According to the Center for Disease Control and Prevention (CDC), heart disease, cancer, stroke, and diabetes cause well over half of all American deaths.[7] Obesity increases the risk for all of them. Treating these chronic illnesses costs billions of dollars to our health care system—and wallets. In 2008, medical costs related to obesity were estimated to be $147 billion.[8] Not to mention, being overweight or obese affects one's livelihood and quality of life.

These statistics are alarming, especially when portion control is one of the easiest ways to manage weight. Controlling portion sizes is right in front of us, with no fancy diet or exercise gadget needed. Tennis players should pay heed to not only what they eat but how much.

The USDA's MyPlate graphic, which replaced the long-standing Food Guide Pyramid in 2011, is now America's nutritional icon.[9] First Lady Michelle Obama unveiled the MyPlate symbol in 2011 to support her Healthy, Hunger-Free Kids Act, part of the Let's Move! national campaign. This campaign enacts legislation to improve the nutritional status of children, simultaneously addressing the overweight and obesity epidemic. MyPlate is a simple graphic providing a clear visual message about plate content.

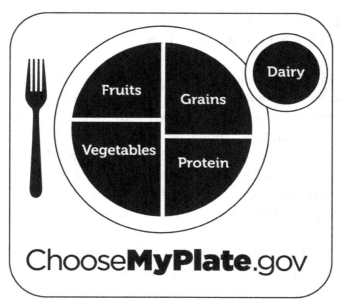

*Graphic 1.1: MyPlate, US Department of Agriculture*

The intent of the recent MyPlate graphic in replacing the long-standing Food Guide Pyramid, first released in 1992 and revised as My Pyramid in 2005, is to provide a single, clear message relating to portion plate allotment when so many conflicting dietary messages are sent through our vast network of information sources. Critics of the Food Guide Pyramid felt it was overcomplicated and difficult to understand.[10] The Food Guide

Pyramid was revised to My Pyramid in 2005 to include a symbol for exercise while its bands were inverted sideways. Still, its many messages may have remained unclear to Americans.

Free from complexities and frills, MyPlate is a simple and straightforward graphic communicating portion control. The MyPlate image suggests that half your eight- to nine-inch meal plate should consist of vegetables and fruits. The remaining quarters of your plate should be assigned to grains and protein. Dairy, a significant provider of calcium, protein, and vitamin D, is close by.

## NATURE'S SUPERFOODS: FRUITS AND VEGETABLES

Epidemiological studies, which evaluate factors influencing the health of populations over a prolonged period of time, have correlated diets high in plant foods with lower rates of obesity, diabetes, cancer, hypertension, heart disease, and stroke. In fact, of all dietary factors in cancer prevention, the most abundant evidence supports the protective effect of fruit and vegetable consumption.[11]

It is no surprise then that half your plate should be covered with fruits and vegetables. This significant plate assignment is worthy of discussion. Fruits and vegetables carry nutritional "bang for the buck." In other words, they are high in nutrition, providing carbohydrates, fiber, and a wide range of vitamins and minerals in the very modest calories they deliver.

Fruits and vegetables also provide phytonutrients, natural plant chemicals (*phyto* = plant). Plant-based foods—such as fruits, vegetables, grains, beans, and tea—contain the most phytonutrients. Animal products—like meat, dairy and eggs—contribute minimal phytonutrients.

Phytonutrients protect plants from environmental damage. There are over twenty-five thousand phytonutrients in plant-based foods. Although they are not essential to life, like vitamins and minerals, scientists propose that certain phytonutrients may prevent the oxidative and inflammatory damage to human cells that lead to cancer and heart disease. Chronic inflammation and cellular oxidation are two of our bodies' response mechanisms to environmental damage. Experts are fervently studying the role of diet, including fruits and vegetables, in reducing chronic inflammation and oxidation.

Fruits and vegetables pack nutritional punch—the makings of a superfood. What's a superfood? Foods coined *superfoods* are named as such because they go beyond basic nutrition and promote superior health in some way. They are usually (but not limited to) whole, unprocessed, natural foods and therefore rarely have a label. Examples of superfoods include certain fruits and vegetables, whole grains, teas, nuts, and seeds. Superfoods are not necessarily plant based. Eggs, yogurt, and certain types of fish have also been labeled superfoods.

There is no legal definition of superfood. Manufacturers may use the term, often loosely, for marketing purposes. Realize a superfood, like most fruits and vegetables, confers superior health benefits.

What's a serving of vegetables and fruits? A one-cup serving of raw vegetables or half-cup serving of cooked vegetables is only twenty-five calories—a bargain for so much nutrition in so few calories. A half- to one-cup serving of fresh fruit is approximately sixty to one hundred calories. The 2010 US Dietary Guidelines recommended eating two and a half cups of vegetables and one and a half cups of fruit per day.

---

**A SERVING OF FRUIT EQUALS THE FOLLOWING:**
- 1 cup of fresh fruit: cut-up melon, strawberries, grapes, pineapple, kiwi
- 1/4 cup of dried fruit: raisins, prunes, dried apricots
- 1 large peach, pear, orange, apple, nectarine
- 1/2 a grapefruit
- 2 medium plums
- 1 medium banana

---

Fruit provides a nutritional profile similar to vegetables, with one exception. The natural sugars present in fruit—glucose and fructose—contribute significantly more calories than the same serving size of vegetables—over twice the amount. If you are watching your caloric and sugar intake, select vegetables more frequently than fruits, or use discretion in portion size when you choose fruits over vegetables.

The USDA MyPlate guidelines classify vegetables into several categories based on their nutritional profile.[12]

---

### CATEGORIES OF VEGETABLES (USDA)
- dark-green vegetables: broccoli, spinach, greens, kale
- red and orange vegetables: carrots, pumpkin, red peppers, tomatoes, and acorn, butternut, and Hubbard squash
- starchy vegetables: corn, green peas, lima beans, potatoes
- beans and peas: black, pinto, kidney, garbanzo, and lentils
- other vegetables: includes the rest of the pack, such as asparagus, cucumber, green beans, eggplant, mushrooms

---

All vegetables are good for you. However, if you can put vegetables on a color continuum, target the ones with deep green, orange, purple, and red pigment. These vegetables are the cream of the crop, meaning they provide the most nutrition of any of the listed categories. Consume the vegetables in categories one and two on a daily basis. (If you are on a blood thinner, consult with your MD or RD about the high vitamin K content in the vegetables in the first category.)

Does that make paler vegetables like potatoes and turnips unhealthy? Of course not. They provide nutrients, vitamins, and minerals too. However, deeply colored vegetables and fruits tend to have more vitamins, like beta-carotene, folic acid, and vitamin C.

The pigment in the more colorful vegetables also has more phytonutrient power believed to prevent disease. Fruits and vegetables have their beautiful colors for a reason. The plant pigments are phytonutrients that protect them from environmental damage and act as antioxidants. Antioxidants protect plant cells from oxidative damage. When we consume foods rich in antioxidants, such as fruits and vegetables, experts theorize their protective benefits apply to the human body too.

Oxidative damage causes disease in humans. Just as oxidation causes a car to rust, oxidative damage harms cells in our bodies. Damaging by-products of oxidation are known as free radicals. Free radicals are formed from environmental elements like pollution or smog (e.g., ozone), as well as smoking, alcohol, and sun exposure (radiation)—environmental elements we can control.

Constant exposure to these damaging environmental elements results in free radical formation in the cells of our bodies. Free radicals are very reactive, unstable atoms or molecules having a single, unpaired electron on their outer surface. Normal, stable atoms always have a pair of electrons on their outer surface. Once formed, unstable free radicals can start a chain reaction, damaging the cell membrane and DNA of healthy cells. DNA is the genetic building block or "blueprint" for cell production.

Antioxidants found in fruits and vegetables may "scavenge" or neutralize these free radicals before they do their oxidative damage to healthy cells. When applied to the human body, this protective action may reduce the risk for diseases, such as cancer and heart disease, still the two top causes of mortality in the United States. Free radicals are also believed to be the cause of accelerated aging.

Oxidative and inflammatory damage to cells are the root causes of major disease. Inflammation is the body's natural response to acute injury or irritants. An acute injury, such as a cut or scrape, elicits an inflammatory response. However, when the irritants keep appearing over and over (as with smoking, poor diet, and stress), the body is in a chronic proinflammatory state, which can damage cells. Chronic inflammation harms, not heals.

Components in our diet, including fruits and vegetables, may reduce the risk of cellular oxidative and inflammatory damage. Of the thousands of antioxidants found in foods, the most potent and beneficial are listed below.

**Table 1.1: Antioxidants in Plant Foods**

| Phytonutrient | Foods Containing |
|---|---|
| **1. Flavonoids**—The flavonoids listed below may decrease risk of cancer and heart disease | |
| Resveratrol | Red grapes, grape juice, red wine<br>Berries: blackberries, blueberries, strawberries, cranberries<br>prunes, plums, pomegranate |
| Catechins | Black and green tea |
| Anthocyanidins | Prunes, plums, acai berry<br>Blueberries, cherries<br>Red, black, and pinto beans |
| Flavonols | Apples, berries, grapes, onions |
| **2. Carotenoids** | |
| Alpha- and beta-carotene—may boost immune function | Carrots, sweet potato, pumpkin<br>Leafy greens: kale, spinach<br>Broccoli<br>Peaches, cantaloupe, apricots |
| Lycopene—linked to reduction of prostate cancer | Tomato and tomato products<br>Watermelon, pink grapefruit |
| Lutein and zeaxanthin—helps protect against cataracts and age-related macular degeneration | Spinach, kale, dandelion greens<br>Turnip and collard greens, corn<br>Egg yolks, nuts (pistachio) |
| **3. Vitamin C**—boosts immune function and prevents infection | Citrus fruits: oranges, grapefruit, tangerines, orange juice<br>Strawberries, bell peppers, kiwi |

| Phytonutrient | Foods Containing |
|---|---|
| 4. Vitamin E—possibly reduces risk of cancer and heart disease (recent study is controversial) | Whole grains, nuts (almonds, peanuts, hazelnuts), sunflower seeds, vegetable oils, wheat germ |
| 5. Minerals | |
| Selenium—trace element may help prevent certain cancers | Brazil nuts, organ and muscle meats, seafood, cereals, and grains |
| 6. Isoflavones—genistein and daidzein may reduce risk of prostate and breast cancer | Soy foods: edamame, tofu, soy milk, tempeh, soy nuts |

Although there are still conflicting findings on the therapeutic effect of specific phytonutrients, the evidence supporting the tremendous health benefits of consuming plant-based foods is overwhelming—so convincing that many experts promote consuming nine servings of fruits and vegetables a day.[13] Almost all leading health organizations recommend consuming a minimum of five servings of vegetables and fruits per day, specifically two servings of fruit and three servings of vegetables. This amount ensures that you are getting their power-packed nutritional benefit. For an individualized recommendation based on your age, gender, and activity level, log on to the CDC's fruit and vegetable calculator (cdc.gov/nutrition/everyone/fruitsvegetables/index.html).

## BENEFITS OF A PLANT-BASED DIET

Many athletes, including tennis players, choose a plant-based or vegetarian diet. These diets all but guarantee that vegetarians consume five to nine servings of vegetable and fruits each day. Along with adequate protein through plant sources (such as beans, peas, legumes, nuts, nut butters, and soy), the health benefits of a plant-based diet are strikingly convincing. The Academy of Nutrition and Dietetics 2009 position paper on the vegetarian diet touts its benefits in both prevention and even reversal of symptoms related to America's most common diseases, including type 2 diabetes, cardiovascular disease, and some types of cancer. These experts proclaim that

> vegetarian diets, including total vegetarian or vegan diets, are healthful, nutritionally adequate, and may provide health benefits in the prevention and treatment of certain diseases. Well-planned vegetarian diets are appropriate for individuals at all stages of the life cycle, including pregnancy, infancy, childhood and adolescence, and for athletes.[14]

A well-planned vegetarian diet is suitable for athletes, including tennis players. If you are considering going meatless, consult with an RD first to determine an eating plan that includes adequate calories, protein, fat, and vitamins and minerals your active tennis body needs.

If you are thinking about going vegan but feel it is too drastic of a jump from your conventional animal protein–based diet, try a gradual shift. Many vegetarians follow a lacto-ovo diet that is less restrictive than a vegan diet—a logical transition to a full plant-based vegan diet.

---

**CLASSIFICATIONS OF VEGETARIAN DIETS:**
- lacto-ovo-vegetarian diet—includes milk and eggs
- lacto-vegetarian diet—includes milk only
- ovo-vegetarian diet—includes eggs only
- pecto-vegetarian diet—includes milk, eggs, and fish
- vegan—includes plant-based foods only and excludes all animal products
- semivegetarian or flexitarian diet—a newer class of vegetarians who eat eggs, dairy, and small amounts of animal protein

---

Many organizations, including the Physicians Committee for Responsible Medicine (PCRM), have improvised the USDA's MyPlate, using their own symbol to promote the plant-based diet. Their PowerPlate is based on the vegan diet, supported by hundreds of studies associating its use with lower rates of obesity, hypertension, heart disease, type 2 diabetes, and some cancers—again, the major contributors of morbidity and mortality in the United States. The PowerPlate has four plant-based meal sections on its plate: fruits, grains, legumes, and vegetables.[15]

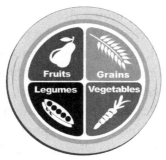

*Graphic 1.2: PowerPlate, Physicians Committee for Responsible Medicine*

## STATE OF OUR PLATE: WHERE ARE THE VEGETABLES?

Whether choosing MyPlate or the PowerPlate, America's plates are not nearly meeting the daily recommendation of five to nine servings of vegetables and fruits per day. According to the Center for Disease Control and Prevention's 2009 analysis, only 14 percent of Americans consume five or more servings of vegetables and fruits per day.[16] Even more concerning is the CDC's report that only 9.5 percent of teens consume five or more servings of vegetables and fruit per day.[17] More than likely, fruits and vegetables are being replaced by other less desirable foods: chips, candy, fast food, and sugary beverages would be no surprise.

Before you try a new diet or supplement, ask yourself if you are getting the unsurpassed nutrition from at least five servings of vegetables and fruit each day. Adults, teens, and children all need to make concerted effort to increase vegetables and fruit in their diet. Incorporate some or all the following tips to get the tremendous health benefits of vegetables and fruit:

1. **Salads.** Precut lettuce of all varieties, spinach, kale, and other raw vegetables, such as carrots, grape tomatoes, peppers, cauliflower, and broccoli, make it easy to prepare nutrition-packed salads. Toss on edamame, garbanzo beans, quinoa, or brown rice for a supernutritious meal. Up to three servings of vegetables or more can be achieved through salad, making it a delicious and efficient way to get the nutritional benefits of vegetables. Along with some healthy protein from whole grains, legumes, nuts, and beans, salads can be a nutritionally power-packed meal. Use a vinegar and oil-based (preferably canola, walnut, sesame, or extra-virgin olive oil) salad dressing, and forego high sodium, saturated/polyunsaturated fat-laden creamy ones. Salad bars and fresh ready-made salads make eating vegetables more convenient for tennis players on the go.

2. **Whole fruit.** There is a reason tennis players of all ranks pull out a banana from their tennis bags. Bananas, grapes, oranges, apples, peaches, pears—these are a few examples of whole fruits that provide carbohydrates, vitamins, minerals, fiber, and phytonutrients in a convenient package. Dried fruit (such as raisins, apples, cherries, goji berries, cranberries, and apricots) also make a healthy and delicious snack.

3. **In recipes.** Substitute or add fruits and vegetables to your favorite recipes. Add carrots, eggplant, corn, kale—any of your favorite vegetables—to soups, chili, and side dishes. Berries, cantaloupe, and honeydew make an excellent base

for refreshing chilled soups—a nice change of pace for post-tennis refreshment.

4. **Replace a high-sugar, high-fat dessert with fruit.** Using fruits you have not tried before will add more interest to dessert and is a good way of expanding variety. If you must curb your craving for something sweet, reach for fruit. Eating sweet desserts like cakes, cookies, pie, and pastries is a learned behavior; you can reteach your brain to be satisfied with a piece of fruit rather than a piece of fruit pie.

   If fruit alone will still not satisfy a sweet tooth, eat a smaller portion of your favorite dessert and accompany it with a portion of fresh fruit like antioxidant-rich berries. Berries, high in fiber, vitamins, and antioxidants, reign supreme as the near-perfect fruit. A four-ounce portion of chocolate mousse, pudding, ice cream, sorbet, or crème brûlée with a large side of fresh raspberries, blueberries, and/or blackberries are decadent desserts earning nutritional merit from fresh fruit.

5. **Drink them.** Toss your favorite fresh or frozen fruits and vegetables in a blender, juicer, or the popular "bullet" mixer for nutrient-rich smoothies or juice. You can achieve a number of servings of fruits and vegetables in one large glass of juice. Nutrient-rich vegetables that you may normally not choose to eat alone (like kale, spinach, or swiss chard) can be tossed in the juicer. These leafy greens are chock-full of vitamins, minerals, and phytonutrients.

   Since the fibrous structure of the fruit and vegetable is broken down, the one drawback of juicing is the reduction in fiber from the otherwise whole fruit or vegetable. Also, be wary of the calories that can add up by juicing fruits. Two or three whole pieces of fruit, along with juice, can easily add up to well over 250 calories. Caloric sweeteners like honey, turbinado and agave also bump up the calories.

Be cognizant of what and how much you are adding to your blender to keep your smoothie from delivering portion distortion.

6. **Use them in sauces, salad dressings, and salsas.** Replace high-fat cream sauces with vegetable- or fruit-based sauces, salad dressings, pestos, and salsas to brighten up your main entrée or side dish. Tomato sauce, high in the antioxidant lycopene, wins hands down on pasta compared to high-fat, high-calorie Alfredo or other cream-based sauces. A half-cup portion of mango or pineapple salsa counts as a serving. Lime, orange, and grapefruit juice provide a refreshing substitute for vinegar (acid) in salad dressings. Puree fresh berries to make a delicious raspberry or strawberry vinaigrette dressing. Squeeze the pungent juice of a blood orange into your next homemade vinaigrette dressing.

7. **As a main dish.** Eggplant Parmesan, portobello mushroom burgers, quinoa-stuffed peppers, white bean chili, and homemade veggie burgers are delicious meatless entrées. The creative list goes on. Replacing an animal-based meal with one vegetarian meal or more per week is a simple way to increase vegetables while promoting health.

## CANNED, FROZEN, OR FRESH: WHICH IS THE BEST?

Most people think canned or frozen vegetables and fruit take the backseat to their fresh counterparts. Not so true. Aside from being low cost and available all season, canned and frozen vegetables and fruits may have more nutritional benefit than once believed. Canned fruits and vegetables also make it easier for tennis players on the go to get their daily dose.

Nutrients in such canned vegetables as carrots, corn, and tomatoes have been shown to have higher phytonutrient content when compared to their fresh products. Canned tomatoes, tomato paste, and tomato sauce have a higher lycopene content than fresh tomatoes. Lycopene is the carotenoid pigment and phytonutrient found in tomatoes, which may protect against heart disease and certain cancers. Canned carrots are more easily digestible than their crunchy fresh counterpart, making their beta-carotene phytonutrients more available for use by the body.

Contrary to what many consumers think, nutrients in canned vegetables and fruits may also be more stable than in fresh produce. Canned and frozen vegetables are picked and processed at their peak. Despite processing, the majority of their nutrients remain. In contrast, fresh vegetables can gradually lose their nutrition from the time they are picked, shipped, purchased, and stored over a period of several days. Spinach can quickly lose its vitamin C when left in the refrigerator for days. Canned or frozen versions may be more nutritious than fresh vegetables stored over a prolonged period of time, when their nutrients can be destroyed. For this reason, use fresh produce as soon as possible, when its nutritional value is at its peak.

Be wary of the salt and sugar content of canned vegetables and fruits. Choose low-salt, no-salt, and low-sugar varieties of canned vegetables and fruits. The added salt in vegetables can transform a naturally low-sodium food to a high-sodium one. Peaches or pears swimming in heavy syrup become high in refined, added sugars. Choose canned fruit packed in its own juice, water, or natural fruit juice.

## ORGANIC OR NONORGANIC: WHICH ONE PREVAILS?

Discriminating produce consumers choose to buy organic fruits and vegetables for reasons that vary depending on their personal, philosophical, and environmental beliefs. I know many health-conscious tennis players who swear by their organic produce. What does *organic* mean? Organic farming requires farmers to use environmentally friendly practices, such as soil management, crop rotation, and pest control and fertilization methods free of chemically manufactured products, such as synthetic pesticides. Organic farming does not incorporate genetically modified organisms (GMOs). Organic operations must maintain or enhance soil or water quality while conserving wetlands, woodlands, and wildlife. Producers and handlers of organic food must be certified and comply with standards set by the government.[18]

There are obvious pros and cons to buying organic produce. Organic produce has lower pesticide residues than conventionally grown produce. The common drawback to consumers is the extra expense of organic produce compared to conventionally grown produce. Are the pesticide residues on conventionally grown fruits and vegetables high enough to warrant the extra dollars spent on organic produce? It depends upon what's tolerable to you.

Pesticide residues are found in our bodies when we consume foods grown with these chemicals. The Environmental Protection Agency (EPA) reports the pesticide levels used on produce are safe at tolerable limits—as with any substance, good or bad, it is about the amount we are exposed to that makes the impact. As an analogy, we know ultraviolet (UV) rays from sun exposure are not good for skin; however, does it mean we stay indoors under the covers at all times to hide from this harmful radiation? Of course not. We make an effort to limit our exposure and take actions to protect ourselves by wearing sunscreen, protective clothing, and sunglasses.

As with minimizing UV exposure, the same can be done with reducing exposure to pesticide residues. Proper washing and scrubbing of fruits and vegetables reduce the chemicals found in conventionally grown produce. Be wary of commercial fruit-and-vegetable rinses and detergents, as their residues left on produce can be suspect for their safety, even more than the pesticide residues they aim to scrub away.

If the thought of having pesticide residues in your food makes you squirm and you question the concept of EPA's tolerable limits, then spending more on organic produce may be your comfortable choice. Many consumers purchase a combination of both organic and conventionally grown produce. There is a basis for this, thanks to the work done by the Environmental Work Group (EWG).

EWG releases its "Shoppers Guide to Pesticides in Produce" to help consumers discern the pesticide content in organic and conventionally grown produce. EWG compiles the list of its "dirty dozen" and "clean fifteen." The "dirty dozen" is the list of commonly purchased fruits and vegetables containing the highest pesticide load, while the "clean fifteen" lists the produce with the lowest pesticide load. This review is based on an analysis of forty-eight most popular fruits and vegetables, with over twenty-eight thousand samples tested by USDA and Food and Drug Administration (FDA) labs.[19]

**Table 1.2: Environmental Working Group's (EWG) Dirty Dozen and Clean Fifteen Lists (Source: Executive Summary, EWG's Shoppers Guide to Pesticides in Produce, 2014)**

| Dirty Dozen (most pesticide residues) | Clean Fifteen: (fewest pesticide residues) |
|---|---|
| 1. Apples | 1. Avocados |
| 2. Strawberries | 2. Sweet Corn |
| 3. Grapes | 3. Pineapples |
| 4. Celery | 4. Cabbage |
| 5. Peaches | 5. Sweet Peas (frozen) |
| 6. Spinach | 6. Onions |
| 7. Sweet Bell Peppers | 7. Asparagus |
| 8. Nectarines (imported) | 8. Mangoes |
| 9. Cucumbers | 9. Papaya |
| 10. Cherry Tomatoes | 10. Kiwi |
| 11. Snap Peas (imported) | 11. Eggplant |
| 12. Potatoes | 12. Grapefruit |
| | 13. Cantaloupe |
| | 14. Cauliflower |
| | 15. Sweet Potatoes |

If apples, grapes, spinach, and strawberries are a few of your produce mainstays, consider using the organic alternative. They are probably worth paying the extra money for, especially if you have children in the house. Children have much smaller bodies and higher metabolisms than grown-ups; therefore, the concentrations of pesticides from fruits and vegetables can be much higher in their body tissues than in those of adults. Children can also be picky eaters, often eating the same fruits and vegetables—apples being a very popular one. By doing so, they are repeatedly exposed to the same pesticide, placing a potentially higher toxicity level in their small bodies.

The American Academy of Pediatrics (AAP) agrees that the level of pesticide residues in organic produce may be significant for children, since they are uniquely vulnerable to chemical exposure.[20] The AAP endorses use of shoppers guides, like EWG's, as references for parents when making decisions on buying conventionally grown versus organic produce.

Produce that has met USDA requirements to be certified organic is distinguished by their characteristic seal. This seal signifies that certified organic produce is free of synthetic fertilizers, pesticides, sewage sludge, ionizing radiation, and genetically modified organisms. Certified organic meat and poultry is free of antibiotics and growth hormones.[21] By growing organically, farmers focus on renewable resources and conservation of soil and water to promote environmental sustainability. Many states and local farms also have their own various, unique certification seals or stamps on their organic produce.

Whether organic or conventionally grown, there is no clear evidence to date that organic produce is more nutritious than conventionally grown produce.[22] However, there is evidence pointing to the direction that organic produce may be healthier because it is free of pesticides that were registered as safe by the EPA long before further research was done to link these chemicals with cancer, attention deficit hyperactivity disorder (ADHD), and other diseases.[23] More research needs to be done to prove this theory.

Most recent study also suggests that organic produce has higher antioxidant content than nonorganic produce. In a 2014 study published in the *British Journal of Nutrition*, researchers found that organic fruits, vegetables, and cereals contained higher concentrations of antioxidants than conventionally grown produce and a lower content of toxic metals and pesticides. This study established the compositional differences between organic and nonorganic produce, a starting point to help quantify the health impacts of organic produce.[24]

While half your plate should be covered with colorful vegetables and fruits, one-quarter of the plate should consist of grains. Grains provide carbohydrates, fiber, iron, and B vitamins. Many grains also provide phytonutrients. (Chapter 5, which presents an in-depth review of carbohydrates, discusses the beneficial nutrition in grains.)

The final quarter of your plate should include your protein source. If choosing animal-based sources of protein, like beef, pork, lamb, and chicken, keep the portion in control. In general, animal sources of protein should contribute about three ounces per cooked serving, the equivalent of twenty-one grams of protein in a serving.

This amount is significantly smaller than restaurant-sized portions or the portion you may be used to cooking at home or choosing at the tennis venue. A three-ounce portion of cooked meat is the size and thickness of a deck of playing cards—a far cry from the mammoth sixteen-ounce T-bone steak commonly served at the neighborhood steak house. (Chapter 3 discusses protein in detail.)

## TENNIS PLAYERS NEED CALCIUM, VITAMIN D, AND PHOSPHOROUS

A symbol for dairy is adjacent to the plate, representing milk or yogurt to supply calcium, phosphorous, and vitamin D. Keep in mind that these nutrients can come from other sources besides dairy. They include fortified orange juice; soy, almond, cashew, oat, hemp, and rice milk and the products made from these sources; and a select few calcium-containing vegetables, such as collard greens, bok choy, spinach, okra, and kale.

These nutrients are necessary throughout all stages of the life span for normal bone growth and development. Active tennis players need them to keep bones strong. Bones support muscles and protect organs. Strong bones are not only necessary for peak tennis performance but to keep your body safe from injury on and off the court.

Calcium, vitamin D, and phosphorous are essential nutrients for bone health and disease prevention. Osteomalacia is the reduction of bone density, which can lead to greater risk of fractures—at any stage in life. Bone density is used to describe the bone after the developmental period is completed, while bone mass refers to bone mineral content accumulated prior to cessation of growth.[25]

Osteoporosis is the age-related decrease in bone mass, which can also be caused by calcium and vitamin D deficiency along with age-related losses, particularly after menopause in women, when estrogen levels decline. Other risk factors for osteoporosis include race (white or people of Asian descent are at higher risk), family history, small or petite body-frame size, sedentary lifestyle, excessive alcohol and tobacco use, hyperthyroidism, and long-term use of corticosteroid medication.

This loss of bone mass results in the inability of bones to sustain ordinary strains, making both men and women more susceptible to fractures, particularly later in life. Although osteoporosis is most common in postmenopausal women, men are susceptible to this disease too. After the age of forty, both men and women experience a loss of bone mass. Because of the decrease in estrogen production caused by menopause, women have a significant decline in bone mass after the age of fifty. Men lose bone mass at a much slower rate than women, until the age of seventy when both genders lose bone mass at approximately the same rate.

Many men play tennis well into their seventies, eighties, and even nineties! In order to ensure bone health in these golden years, men also need to choose a diet adequate in calcium, vitamin D, and phosphorous. Because many men think osteoporosis is gender biased toward women, they may ignore bone health along with the inclusion of these important nutrients.

Osteoporosis is the primary culprit for hip and wrist fractures in women and men. Slips and falls, more commonly occurring at older age, will cause fractures when the bones are weak and brittle. Playing the wonderful sport of tennis well into our golden years does make us more vulnerable to falls. Even after rehabilitation, the damage done by fractures can be irreparable to our return to the tennis court.

Like calcium, vitamin D is also an essential nutrient for bone health. Vitamin D regulates calcium absorption and maintains phosphorous levels in the blood. Most commonly associated with its role in bone heath, recent research suggests vitamin D may also have other important functions. Vitamin D may enhance immune function and reduce exercise-related inflammation. There is current research on the role of Vitamin D in prevention of cancer, particularly colon and rectal cancer.[26]

The body produces vitamin D through exposure to ultraviolet B light (UVB) in the skin. As UVBs come from sunlight exposure, it is no surprise that vitamin D is nicknamed the "sunshine vitamin." We also get vitamin D through fortified foods in our diet. Because calcium and vitamin D have clear roles in bone health, the Institute of Medicine recently revealed their new recommendations for calcium and vitamin D listed in the table 1.3.[27] With emerging discovery of vitamin D's role beyond bone health, achieving adequate amounts through diet and sunlight exposure are essential.

**Table 1.3: Calcium, Phosphorous, and Vitamin D Requirements (Source: Institute of Medicine, 2009)**

| Category | Calcium (mg/day) | Phosphorous (mg/day) | Vitamin D (IU) |
|---|---|---|---|
| Children | | | |
| 1–3 yr | 700 | 460 | 600 |
| 4–8 yr | 1,000 | 500 | 600 |
| 9–18 yr | 1,300 | 1,250 | 600 |
| 19–70 yr | 1,000 | 700 | 600 |
| 51–70 yr-old males | 1,000 | 700 | 600 |
| 51–70 yr-old females | 1,200 | 700 | 600 |
| >70 yr | 1,200 | 700 | 800 |
| 14–18 yr-old pregnant/ lactating | 1,300 | 1,250 | 600 |
| 19–50 yr-old pregnant/ lactating | 1,000 | 700 | 600 |

Vitamin D status is determined by blood levels of calcitriol, or 25-hydroxyvitamin D. The Institute of Medicine (IOM) has found that 20 ng/ml is the blood level needed for bone health for most individuals. However, no optimal level has been established for athletes. Blood levels of vitamin D and bone density can be screened through your physical exam.

There are no recommendations for amount of sunlight exposure, since such factors as skin pigmentation, geography, and use of sunscreen affect how much UVB radiation skin absorbs. The darker the skin, the more protective against skin cancer but the less UVB radiation absorption for vitamin D conversion in the skin; the lighter the skin, the less protective against skin cancer but the more UVB radiation absorption.

In general, expose your face, arms, and legs to the sun between the hours of 10:00 a.m. and 2:00 p.m. for a total of ten to twenty-five minutes, two to three times per week, without sunscreen, for this brief exposure. For those at high risk of melanoma or skin cancer, check with your physician first. Much of UVB exposure occurs during such daily activities as simply getting in and out of the car or running errands outside the home. The fact that tennis players are regularly outdoors playing in sunny weather helps ensure sunlight exposure.

Vitamin D also comes from food sources. Vitamin D is naturally present in only a few foods. Examples of these foods include salmon, tuna, fish-liver oils, egg yolks and beef. Interestingly, fish-liver oils provide the richest source of naturally occurring vitamin D. Ever take cod-liver oil when you were a child? This is the reason.

Because very few foods contain naturally-occurring vitamin D, this nutrient is added to foods through fortification. Approximately 98 percent of all fluid milk in the United States is voluntarily fortified with vitamin D. However, contrary to popular belief, milk products like yogurt, cottage cheese, and most varieties of hard and soft cheeses are not fortified with vitamin D.[28] Table 1.4 provides the IOM's most recent recommendations for vitamin D intake based on age.[29]

**Table 1.4: Recommended Intake for Vitamin D (Source: Institute of Medicine, 2010)**

| Age | Amount (IU) |
| --- | --- |
| 0–12 months | 400 |
| 1–70 years | 600 |
| >70 years | 800 |

Phosphorous, a mineral-like calcium, also helps build bone and teeth. Phosphorous has many other functions. Phosphorous helps the body use carbohydrates and fat and is essential for muscle contraction, kidney function, and normal heartbeat. The many functions of phosphorous go well beyond bone health. Along with dairy products, phosphorous is found in meat and nuts.

Much of the three bone-building nutrients come from dairy

products. Dairy products are also rich in potassium, carbohydrates, protein, and B vitamins. Skim milk and 1 percent milk are the healthier, low-fat alternatives to whole and 2 percent milk for adults and children over the age of two. Yogurt is also a rich source of calcium and protein. Yogurt and kefir contain live cultures or probiotics. Probiotics support production of "good bacteria" in our gut, essential for digestion and absorption of nutrients.

Dairy products like milk have received unfavorable attention from their nutrition naysayers. There are a number of reasons. One argument is that consuming dairy products from cows is "unnatural," because humans are the only species that consume milk in adulthood and from another animal. Lactose intolerance is the inability of our bodies to break down lactose—the carbohydrate, or sugar, in milk—due to lack of the digestive enzyme lactase. Lactose intolerance causes such symptoms as gas, bloatedness, and diarrhea. Many people are lactose intolerant. In fact, up to 65 percent of the adult world population has reduced ability to digest lactose, causing varying symptoms of lactose intolerance.[30]

Some experts feel that milk and dairy intake are not needed to reduce fractures. They point out that many countries in which almost no milk is consumed, such as Asian countries, have low rates of fractures.

It is also important to know that people do not have to drink milk to be healthy, mostly because milk's nutrition can come from other food sources. There are a number of nondairy foods and beverages that contribute calcium and vitamin D; examples include calcium-fortified orange juice and fortified soy, rice, oat, hemp, and almond milk—popular vegan alternatives to cow's milk. Tofu processed in calcium sulfate is another nondairy source of calcium. Certain green vegetables like collard greens, broccoli, kale, and spinach also provide calcium and vitamin D. However, the calcium in these leafy greens has reduced absorbability compared to milk and dairy products.

What cannot be refuted is the fact that dairy products are

very nutritious. One cup of milk contains about 25 percent of the recommended daily amounts for calcium, vitamin D, riboflavin (vitamin B2), and phosphorous. Add potassium, protein, vitamin B12, zinc, and magnesium to the list and milk starts looking like a superfood. If you enjoy and can tolerate milk and dairy products, their nutritional benefit may outweigh their controversy, making a compelling argument in their favor. Table 1.5 provides the caloric, protein, fat, calcium, and vitamin D content of dairy and nondairy foods.[31]

**Table 1.5: Nutrient Content of Dairy and Nondairy Foods—Per 8 oz. serving, unless specified (Source: USDA National Nutrient Database for Standard Reference, Release 18)**

| | Calories | Fat | Protein | Calcium | Vitamin D |
|---|---|---|---|---|---|
| **Dairy** | | g | g | mg | IU |
| Whole Milk | 150 | 8 | 8 | 250 | 100 |
| 2% Milk | 120 | 5 | 8 | 290 | 100 |
| 1% Milk | 110 | 2 | 8 | 290 | 100 |
| Skim Milk | 90 | 0 | 8 | 300 | 100 |
| Low Fat Chocolate Milk | 140 | 2 | 8 | 300 | 100 |
| Yogurt, Low Fat | 150 | 2 | 9 | 450 | 100 |
| Greek Yogurt, fat-free, 6 oz. | 150 | 0 | 15 | 200 | 0* |
| Cottage Cheese, 1% | 160 | 2 | 25 | 130 | 0* |
| **Nondairy** | | | | | |
| Fortified Orange Juice | 90 | 0 | 0 | 300 | 100 |
| Soy Milk, fortified | 80 | 4 | 10 | 250-300 | 40-120 |
| Almond Milk (sweetened) | 60 | 2.5 | 1 | 450 | 100 |
| Collard Greens (cooked) | 49 | 1 | 4 | 270 | — |
| Tofu (5 oz.), firm | 100 | 5 | 10 | 290 | — |
| Kale (raw) | 33 | 0 | 2 | 55 | — |
| Spinach (cooked) | 41 | 0 | 5 | 240 | — |

Whole milk and 2 percent milk and the cheese, yogurt, and cottage cheese made with these milk sources should be limited due to their higher caloric and saturated fat content. Although of recent dispute, research suggests a high intake of saturated fat over time leads to high blood cholesterol levels, a risk factor linked to heart disease. The one exception supporting consumption of full-fat dairy products is for children under the age of two years; the American Academy of Pediatrics recommends that children under two years old drink whole milk to supply needed calories, fat, and cholesterol for proper growth and development.

To consume the amount of calcium and vitamin D necessary for healthy bones, include low-fat, calcium-rich foods and beverages in your meals every day. For tennis players concerned about calories in dairy products, the Recommended Daily Allowance (RDA) for calcium, vitamin D, and phosphorous can be met in three hundred calories or fewer per day.

## BOOST YOUR CALCIUM, PHOSPHOROUS, AND VITAMIN D INTAKE

Use these tips to boost your calcium and vitamin D intake:

1.  Drink calcium-fortified orange juice. The amount of calcium and vitamin D in one cup of calcium-fortified orange juice is equivalent to the amounts of those nutrients in one cup of skim milk. Orange juice is also high in potassium, folic acid, and vitamin C. Plus, the calcium in orange juice is as absorbable as the calcium in dairy products.

2.  Have cereal and milk for breakfast. Whole-grain cereal with skim, low-fat, or fortified soy milk packs nutritional punch, including a good percentage of the day's calcium requirement. Calcium and vitamin D–fortified almond, oat, hemp, and rice milk are also excellent nondairy

sources. Be sure these nondairy sources are fortified; if not, they do not count as a source of calcium and vitamin D. Since the calcium can settle on the bottom of the container of fortified soy, rice, and almond milk, be sure to shake your carton before each use.

3. Prepare hot cereal, such as oatmeal, soups, and sauces with skim, low-fat, or soy milk. Not only will this enhance the flavor of these foods, but it will provide extra protein, B vitamins, calcium, and vitamin D.

4. Eat yogurt. Yogurt is a near-perfect food, high in protein, potassium, B vitamins, calcium, vitamin D, and probiotics. Greek yogurt is the superstar of yogurts, high in protein and nutrition. Greek yogurt is yogurt that has been strained or filtered to remove excess whey. This straining makes even fat-free varieties of greek yogurt extraordinarily rich and creamy.

5. Add yogurt, milk, soy milk, or calcium-processed tofu to smoothies. Use fresh or frozen fruits and vegetables high in vitamins and antioxidants for nutrient-packed pre- or post-tennis fuel.

6. Use low-fat cheese on quesadillas, salads, and grilled cheese sandwiches. Cheese or veggie pizza made with part-skim mozzarella cheese and an array of veggies can be a nutrient-rich vegetarian meal.

7. Choose calcium-rich desserts, such as frozen yogurt, custard, and pudding. Accompany them with some fresh nutrient-powered berries for an even healthier dessert.

8. Use milk in your coffee or tea rather than cream, sugary flavored creamers with hydrogenated oils, or half-and-half. A mocha latte made with soy or low-fat milk is a calcium-rich treat.

## PROBIOTICS: "GOOD FOR LIFE"

Yogurt also contains active live cultures or probiotics. *Probiotic* means "good for life" for a reason. Probiotics are live microorganisms that provide health benefits when consumed in adequate amounts. Probiotics are found in our digestive tract, where they help digest food and combat pathogens that can be harmful to our bodies.

Probiotics augment the microbial population in our digestive tract, or gut. There are one hundred trillion bacteria in our intestines, much of which is good bacteria, keeping our digestive tract healthy. Because over 65 percent of the cells that make up our immune function are in our gut, probiotics may improve our immunity, working to fight off infection and disease.

Of the approximately five hundred types of bacteria in our gut, there are several that are beneficial to digestive health. *Lactobacillus* bacteria and *Bifidobacteria* are the two most common types of microbes used as probiotics. Both are found in yogurt, containing live and active cultures, and other fermented milk products, such as kefir, which contains even more strains of good bacteria than yogurt. Aged cheeses also contain probiotics. Other less commonly known sources of probiotics include fermented foods like sauerkraut; miso; tempeh; kimchi, a spicy fermented cabbage common in the Korean diet; and kombucha, a fermented beverage made from black and green tea.

Probiotics may be especially useful when a person takes antibiotics. Antibiotics can destroy both the harmful and beneficial bacteria in our digestive tract, causing antibiotic-induced diarrhea. This obliteration of healthy bacteria in our gut can also lead to yeast infections and urinary tract infections. Since the amount recommended during certain antibiotic treatment is high, probiotic supplements may be necessary. Seek guidance from your health care professional if you want to take probiotic supplements during antibiotic treatment.

Not to be confused with probiotics, prebiotics are nondigestible, nonabsorbable carbohydrates or soluble fibers that act as food or "fertilizer" to stimulate the growth of probiotics in the digestive tract. Prebiotics promote growth of probiotics. Prebiotics include fructooligosaccharides (FOS) and inulin. Inulin is an effective prebiotic found in onions, asparagus, garlic, bananas, and jerusalem artichokes. FOS is extracted from the blue agave plant, which has one of the highest concentrations of this prebiotic. Prebiotics and probiotics from foods we eat have a mutualistic relationship, working together to promote digestive health.

Prebiotics and probiotics are analogous to a doubles tennis team, working together in winning tandem. Eating foods with prebiotics and probiotics together is ideal. Foods that combine prebiotics and probiotics are called synbiotics. Examples of synbiotics, food components working synergistically, include the following:

- yogurt with sliced bananas
- stir-fried tempeh, asparagus, garlic, and onion
- banana and kombucha
- double-aged gouda or cheddar cheese slices with a side of asparagus and artichoke salad in vinaigrette dressing

## MANAGING PORTION DISTORTION

The MyPlate symbol appears to show the plate sections covered with food, with the potentially misunderstood message that your entire plate must be full to meet nutritional requirements. An entire plate does not need to be filled to the rim with food to fulfill nutritional needs.

Fortunate to live in this land of plenty, we may be tainted with the "more is better" mentality about food. Over the years, marketing studies show that portion sizes of almost every imaginable food item have increased, in some cases unabashedly "supersized."[32] Our culture certainly promotes "the bigger the better" adage when it comes to portion sizes.

According to the National Heart, Lung, and Blood Institute (NHLBI), average portion sizes on certain foods compared to twenty years ago have doubled, even tripled, in size and calories.[33] Twenty years ago, a muffin used to be about the size of an egg and contain 210 calories. Today, a typical muffin has morphed into a softball-sized, megabreakfast at 500 calories. Soft drinks in twenty-ounce bottles are still not big enough, with fast-food restaurants and convenience stores supersizing them into forty-eight-ounce barrels. Ironically, several beverage distributors have gone retro, shrinking a twelve-ounce can to eight ounces, considered "petite" versions by our today's portion standard while they are still as big as twenty years ago! Children, teens, and adults do not need the excess calories, sugar, fat, and sodium in these large portions. Table 1.6 outlines further comparison of portion sizes twenty years ago and today.

**Table 1.6: Portion Sizes Twenty Years Ago and Today (Source: National Heart, Lung, and Blood Institute)**

|  | Twenty Years Ago | | Today | |
| --- | --- | --- | --- | --- |
| Item | Portion | Calories | Portion | Calories |
| Bagel | 3-inch diameter | 140 | 6-inch diameter | 280 |
| Soda | 6.5 oz. | 85 | 20 oz. | 240 |
| Pizza, pepperoni | 1 slice | 250 | 2 slices | 500 |
| Muffin | 1.5 oz. | 210 | 4.5 oz. | 500 |

Repeated studies show we respond to increased portion sizes by eating more. Even when we are satiated, we still eat more when there is more on our plate and drink more when there is more in our cup or bottle. Barbara Rolls, PhD, professor of nutritional science at Penn State University and founder of the Volumetrics diet, has observed this with men, women, dieters, nondieters, and children.[34]

This portion distortion has plagued consumers of all ages. Portion distortion has brainwashed Americans into thinking that large portions are the norm, while they actually provide far too many unneeded calories. Evidently, consuming these excessive calories has contributed to the current, complicated overweight and obesity public health crisis in the United States.

Combined with the common "waste not, want not" attitude, overeating large portions of food makes overweight and obesity an inevitable yet avoidable catastrophe. How many times were you told to clean your full plate by eating every morsel of food? Consuming all the food on your plate is reasonable when the portion size on the plate starts off being reasonable. For the readers who are parents, send the right message on portion control to your children: that good nutrition is foremost about quality, not quantity—which means being prudent about portion sizes.

Use these helpful resources to find a portion-size guide right for you. Many of the sites have portion guides for both adults and kids:

1. http://www.webmd.com/dtmcs/live ... /site ... /portion-control-guide.pdf—helps size food portions to common relatable household items
2. http://www.theportionplate.com/—portion-size plate for omnivores, adult, and children
3. http://www.theveganrd.com/food-guide-vegans—portion-size plate for vegans
4. http://www.health.harvard.edu.healtheatingplate—Harvard Healthy Eating Plate from the Harvard School of Public Health

5. http://www.preciseportions.com—a variety of attractive plates, cups, bowls, utensils, and placemat kits providing healthy eating tips and portion-size guidance

## YOUR PLATE REVISITED

MyPlate indicates the protein portion of the plate should come from an animal source, such as chicken, beef, eggs, pork, or fish—since grains and vegetables, alternate protein sources themselves, have their own plate assignment. Animal sources of protein continue to be the most commonly consumed protein source in the American diet but are certainly not the only sources.

Good sources of protein come from a variety of plant-based foods. Whole grains, legumes, beans, tofu, nuts, and nut butters are all excellent sources of plant protein. These sources of plant protein are not visually represented on USDA's MyPlate. Plant-based sources of protein can contribute a larger portion on your plate, particularly if grains are part of the protein source.

Plant-based vegan diets have been shown to reduce risk of cancer compared to other dietary patterns. In a recent study, epidemiologists found vegan diets to have significant protection for overall cancer incidence when other such factors as weight, gender, and smoking were controlled for.[35] Still keep that section of vegetable-based protein to half or less of the plate coverage. Refer to the PowerPlate on page 15, which depicts what your vegan plate should look like.

Another assumption of the MyPlate recommendation is that milk should be the choice of beverage during meal times. As previously discussed, milk is an important contributor of calcium, phosphorous, vitamin D, and protein in our diet. Milk is a nutritious beverage, which provides nutrients essential to bone health. However, if our diet contains adequate calcium, phosphorous, and vitamin D through other food or beverage sources, milk need not be the beverage of choice. Water is the best alternative at the dinner table when these nutrient needs are met from other sources.

Experts from the Harvard School of Public Health and Harvard Medical School have recently created the Healthy Eating Plate prototype of USDA's MyPlate. The Healthy Eating Plate encourages consumers to choose "healthy protein" sources like fish, poultry, beans, or nuts. It also distinguishes the use of "whole grains" versus "grains" and encourages water as the mealtime beverage of choice. Vegetables occupy a larger plate section than fruits, their higher-sugar counterparts. The Healthy Eating Plate depicts a bottle of healthy oil, like olive or canola oil, for use on salads and bread as opposed to butter or trans fat–laden stick margarine. The intent is to show that choosing healthy oils is beneficial—focusing on the quality of fat, not the quantity. The Harvard Healthy Eating Plate is an excellent prototype to the USDA's MyPlate graphic.[36]

While the USDA's MyPlate may have a few caveats, it sends a vivid nutrition message relatable to all age groups. Because the MyPlate graphic is nutrition policy for all Americans, it innately does not address individualized eating plans. To assist in customizing your daily eating plan, refer to the USDA's official website for MyPlate: www.choosemyplate.gov. This resource provides daily food plans and SuperTracker, a tool that helps plan, analyze, and track your diet and physical activity—individualized for you.

There are also a countless number of diet, nutrition, and fitness apps and devices. Phone apps are great tools to help track and monitor diet and exercise goals. Wrist devices have become very popular diet-, sleep-, and fitness-tracking bracelets. They even provide coaching and advice based on your fitness and nutrition needs.

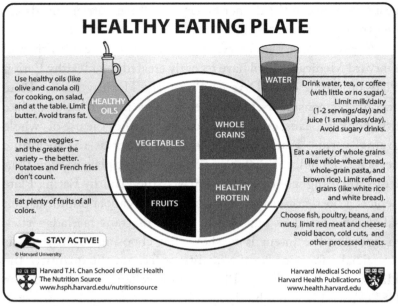

Graphic 1.3: *Harvard Healthy Eating Plate, Harvard University Copyright © 2011, Harvard University. For more information about the Healthy Eating Plate, please see the Nutrition Source, Department of Nutrition, Harvard School of Public Health, www.thenutritionsource. org, and Harvard Health Publications, www.health.harvard.edu.*

Remember Alan at the beginning of the chapter? Alan needs to lose weight sensibly by getting good nutrition in the right amount of calories through a variety of foods to support both his weight management and active tennis lifestyle. Variety in food choices ensures achievement of a wide range of nutrients.

An obvious plus for Alan's weight-loss effort is that he stays active with tennis—singles tennis to boot. But in order to maintain his high energy level during matches, he needs to include the proper balance of a long list of nutrients—carbohydrates, protein, fat, fluids, fiber, phytonutrients, and vitamins and minerals—to ensure peak tennis performance while still getting lean and fit at the same time.

# 2

## SUPPLEMENTS: TO TAKE OR NOT TO TAKE?

**You have to believe in yourself when no one else does—that makes you a winner right there.**
—Venus Williams

Andrea, a local club tennis player, seems to be the picture of health. Like clockwork, she meticulously arranges her colorful supplement pills in the compartments of her organizer, carefully timing her dosages throughout the day. Andrea drinks her wheatgrass smoothie every morning before her three-mile jog. She is 88 percent of her ideal weight with a body mass index (BMI) of seventeen, representing a lean albeit underweight physique. She works out at the gym five times a week, eats a vegan diet, and drinks plenty of fluids. Smoking and drinking alcohol are taboo. But does Andrea represent the picture of health? Not quite. On the tennis courts, Andrea laments. She never felt she had the strength or stamina to carry out her singles matches to the final deciding tiebreak. It turns out Andrea was too "in control"—she overused supplements without getting the adequate calories from the carbohydrates, protein, and fat for these supplements to work on, let alone sustain her active lifestyle. Following professional advice, she whittled her long list of supplements down to a shorter one that made sense. Once she added more calories from a variety of foods, including those with protein and fat, she had more energy, attained a healthier weight, and had the substrates for her supplements to work on.

## SUPPLEMENTS DEFINED

The nutritional supplement industry has exploded in popularity, intrigue, and demand. Manufacturers market and sell supplements to eager consumers at every imaginable corner of the merchandising world. There are many reasons athletes use supplements, but their primary goal is to reap health benefits from supplements or ergogenic aids that they feel they cannot obtain with diet alone.

A dietary supplement is any product that contains substances like vitamins, minerals, foods, botanicals, or amino acids intended to supplement the intake of food in our diet. The International Society of Sports Nutrition (ISSN) describes an ergogenic aid as any training or psychological technique, mechanical device, nutritional practice, or pharmacological agent that can improve exercise performance or physical strength.[37] An ergogenic aid can be a dietary supplement. Many athletes use dietary supplements to give them the competitive edge.

A dietary supplement can be any of the following:

1. **Vitamins.** Vitamins are compounds essential in very small amounts to support normal bodily functions like growth, development, and healing. The body cannot produce these compounds in adequate amounts to keep up with our

needs; therefore, it is essential we get vitamins from the foods we eat.

In the absence of these essential nutrients, vitamin deficiencies occur. Since we now know so much about vitamins, deficiency diseases that were once common in the past are now eradicated with adequate vitamin intake in developed nations. Diseases like rickets, beriberi, pellagra, and scurvy are just about extinct in developed countries because of diet, vitamin supplementation, and fortification of food. Of concern, there has been a slight increase in children with rickets. This may affect children who stay indoors too much, getting inadequate sunlight exposure for their bodies to make vitamin D.[38]

There are two categories of vitamins. They include the fat-soluble vitamins: A, D, E, and K; and the water-soluble vitamins: C, thiamin (vitamin B1), riboflavin (vitamin B2), niacin (vitamin B3), pyridoxine (vitamin B6), cobalamin (vitamin B12), folic acid, biotin, and pantothenic acid. Fat-soluble vitamins are stored in the liver and body tissues. Taking too many fat-soluble vitamins can lead to toxicity. In contrast, excess amounts of water-soluble vitamins are not stored in body tissue but eliminated in urine.

While the essential role of vitamins is well established, understanding their functional role in disease prevention is a contemporary and emerging field. As an example, experts continue to explore the potential antioxidant role that vitamins A, C, and E play in heart disease and cancer prevention. Only recently did scientists discover that folic acid supplementation prior to and during pregnancy prevents disabling neural tube diseases, such as spina bifida. Many people take vitamins for their functional role beyond their essential role.

2. **Minerals.** Minerals are elements that originate in the soil that, like vitamins, cannot be produced by our bodies and must be obtained from food. Minerals come directly from plant sources, such as fruits, vegetables, and grains, and indirectly from animal sources, such as meat, poultry, and seafood. Drinking water also contains minerals. Minerals can vary in food sources, because the mineral content in soil varies in geographic areas.

   Minerals represent 4–5 percent of our body weight. Examples of minerals include calcium (which comprises half the total minerals in our bodies), phosphorous, sodium, potassium, chloride, magnesium, selenium, manganese, fluoride, choline, iron, iodine, chromium, zinc, and copper. Though needed in very small amounts, trace minerals are essential. Believe it or not, we cannot survive without having adequate amounts of copper in our diet, along with a long list of other essential minerals.

3. **Herbs or other botanicals.** Wheatgrass, echinacea, gingko biloba, beetroot juice, and valerian root are only a few examples of botanicals available at the corner grocery or drugstore. The list goes on. Plants have been widely used for their medicinal purposes for thousands of years. Many current prescription and nonprescription drugs are derived from plants. The exploration of plant chemicals will continue to reveal new discoveries in both pharmaceuticals and dietary supplementation.

4. **Amino acids.** Protein is comprised of a variety of amino acids. Specific amino acids serve various functions. Amino acid supplementation is most commonly used for building and repairing muscle tissue before and after workouts. (Amino acids are discussed in detail in chapter 3.)

5. **Other.** The FDA categorizes anything that does not fit in the above classification as "other." This category includes any substance to supplement the diet by increasing total

daily intake—a concentrate, a metabolite, an extract, or any combination of these ingredients. Examples of supplements that do not fall in the first four categories include fish oil capsules, caffeine, and coenzyme Q10. The list in this category is very long too.

## SUPPLEMENTS VERSUS WHOLE FOODS: WHICH IS BETTER?

Experts agree that choosing foods containing naturally occurring nutrients, vitamins, and minerals is best—hands down. Supplements provide the nutrient in chemically isolated form by way of pills, powders, or elixirs. Most studies on supplements have been conducted on animals or humans using the isolated supplement, not the food source of the supplement. Scientists are not sure if isolated, single nutrients or phytochemicals offer the same benefits as those existing synergistically in food sources. Keep that in mind when hearing the latest news or web updates touting the benefits of an isolated nutrient in a pill versus the nutrient from its natural, whole food source.

Even though phytochemicals, like antioxidants, are abundant in fruits and vegetables, their activity, like with all nutrients, depends on how much is actually absorbed and available to the body. Bioavailability is the term used to describe the degree to which nutrients in food are ultimately used by our bodies.[39]

There are many natural substances in food that promote (or prevent) the bioavailability of nutrients. Some nutrients have high bioavailability from foods—what we consume is readily absorbed and used by the body. These include carbohydrates, protein, fat, sodium, potassium, and fluoride. Yet components in food can reduce the bioavailability of nutrients. Phytates in whole grains reduce the absorption of minerals, like calcium and phosphorous. Oxalic acid in collard greens and kale reduce their availability of vitamin D.

Whole foods also contain components that may cause other nutrients to be more bioavailable. The heme iron in meat and poultry is absorbed much better than the nonheme iron in plant foods, like spinach. Other nutrients can make another nutrient more bioavailable too. Vitamin C helps absorb iron in foods, enhancing its bioavailability. Having a few slices of tomato, rich in vitamin C, with a lean hamburger patty enhances the absorption of heme iron in red meat. Half a grapefruit or a small glass of vitamin C–rich orange juice will help absorb the iron in a bowl of iron-fortified cereal or a soft-boiled egg for breakfast.

Vitamin D helps absorb calcium and phosphorous. No wonder milk is fortified with vitamin D to enhance the bioavailability of these bone-building minerals. Simply swallowing a supplement with water will not take advantage of the bioavailability of nutrients in these foods.

Whole foods can also provide a range of nutrients—including vitamins, minerals, and fiber—that cannot be obtained from the isolated supplements. No pill, powder, syrup, or elixir could replace the extra nutrition found in the food source. Whole foods may contain other beneficial components that investigators have not yet discovered.

For example, researchers recently found evidence of antioxidant, anti-inflammatory, and anticancer activity in curcumin, the plant pigment in the pungent spice turmeric commonly used in curry. Curcumin has shown preliminary promise in reducing inflammation, easing symptoms of osteoarthritis and rheumatoid arthritis. Turmeric has been used as a traditional medicine in India and Asia to treat a variety of health conditions.

Researchers have piqued inquiry into the many potential health benefits of cinnamon. Since 2000 BC, ancient civilizations have used cinnamon for its medicinal properties. This very familiar spice may confer a number of health benefits. Most notably, cinnamon may lower blood sugar in people with prediabetes and diabetes. Since no high-quality research supports this claim yet, experts have not recommended the use of cinnamon supplements for management of diabetes.[40] However, research continues to reveal promising functional health benefits of common foods in our very own kitchens.

Beetroot juice has received attention for its naturally occurring nitrate content. Sports scientists are especially interested in beetroot juice's ergogenic effect. Dietary nitrate in beetroot—also found in arugula, spinach, and celery—has been shown to enhance physical performance and exercise stamina by improving blood flow and oxygen delivery to muscles.[41] Oxygen is required to oxidize, or "burn," energy for athletic performance—running down baseline shots, serving aces, and approaching the net for a put away all require bursts of energy.

Specifically, in conditions where the availability of oxygen is low, nitrate can be converted to nitric oxide (NO). Nitric oxide reduces the oxygen cost of exercise (i.e., enhances muscle efficiency) through mechanisms fervently being studied by sports scientists. As a result, dietary nitrate supplementation appears to be a promising ergogenic aid in extending time to exercise exhaustion, increasing stamina and athletic performance.[42]

Andrew M. Jones, PhD, conducted a meta-analysis (a review of many similar studies) on nitrate supplementation, nitric oxide levels, and athletic performance. He concluded that dietary nitrate supplementation of five to seven millimoles (mmol) or 0.1 mmol/kg body mass resulted in significant increases in nitric oxide. The physiological effect of increased nitric oxide levels included lower resting blood pressure, reduced lung oxygen uptake, and possibly enhanced exercise tolerance or performance. These observations occurred in as little as three hours after ingesting dietary nitrate through beetroot juice supplementation.[43] About half a liter of beetroot juice or equivalent of high-nitrate foods, such as spinach, celery, and arugula, can provide the same amount that was given to the study subjects in Jones's research review.

The study of nutrition continues to reveal potential functional benefits of foods in our diet—from vegetables and fruits to teas, herbs, oils, and spices. These health and ergogenic benefits should derive from whole foods first.

## SUPPLEMENTS: ARE THEY SAFE?

There are safety considerations when using dietary supplements. Dietary supplements are not under the same FDA regulatory standards as food and over-the-counter and prescription medications. The FDA's Dietary Supplement Health and Education Act of 1994 (DSHEA) places dietary supplements in a special category of "foods" so they are not considered drugs. Supplements that were on the market prior to 1994 are grandfathered into the DSHEA, meaning the manufacturer is not required to submit evidence to substantiate the safety and effectiveness of their supplement.[44] There are hundreds of supplements that were introduced prior to 1994 still available on today's store shelves for purchase and consumption.

In contrast, new dietary ingredients fall under different safety standards. The FDA now requires manufacturers to provide evidence that the supplement is safe and to substantiate health claims prior to introducing the supplement to the market. This standard helps consumers better discern hype from reality and therefore make educated decisions about the effectiveness of the supplements they choose. The FDA places the burden of proof on the manufacturer of the supplement to make sure the supplement is safe before it is marketed. The FDA takes action against any unsafe product *only after* it reaches the market.

What does this mean to you? Even though there are more regulations governing new supplements, their quality, composition, and purity still need to be closely scrutinized at every purchase— especially for athletes like tennis players. Not all manufacturers will adhere to these regulations. Unscrupulous manufacturers may exaggerate results, suppress negative findings, or falsely attribute poor-quality or minimal research to substantiate their claims. Walk into a local vitamin supplement store, and you will continue to find countless health claims about various nutritional supplements without clear evidence or substantiation that they work. These claims can sound too good to be true, enticing even the more-astute tennis player to be a believer.

Further, poor manufacturing practices, limited regulation, and illegal substances disguised as dietary supplements or ergogenic aids can mislead athletes, tennis players included, and in the extreme circumstances can cause them to test positive for banned substances. This is because supplements can be contaminated with prohibited substances if good manufacturing practices (GMPs) are not adhered to. Many Olympians, as well as professional and collegiate-level athletes, have tested positive for illegal substances found in contaminated dietary supplements.[45]

The International Tennis Federation (ITF) recommends that players be cautious about dietary supplements, since they may contain prohibited substances or be taken in amounts that are not sanctioned.[46] The World Anti-Doping Agency (WADA), which manages the International Olympic Committee's doping control policy, routinely updates its prohibited list of drugs and supplements for athletes. WADA's mission statement is twofold: to protect the athlete and the integrity of the sport.[47]

The US Pharmocopeia (USP) is a nonprofit, third-party organization that sets the standards for identity, purity, quality, and strength of dietary supplements (and drugs) distributed worldwide. The USP's Dietary Supplement Verification Program evaluates dietary supplement contents, manufacturing processes, and compliance with purity standards. USP applies these standards for testing when manufacturers of supplements voluntarily issue their supplements to USP for review.[48]

To reiterate, seeking USP verification for the safety of their supplement is voluntary—not a requirement—for manufacturers. Many manufacturers do not seek to have their products evaluated for safety and purity. If the manufacturer voluntarily verifies their supplement has upheld USP's safety specifications, their product earns the USP designation of quality and safety on the supplement label. Look for the brown, yellow, and black USP stamp on the supplement container.

Other leading organizations have taken steps to ensure the safety of supplements. NSF International, a third-party, global, independent safety watchdog organization certifies the quality, purity, and safety of dietary supplements, as well as other consumer products. NSF International verifies supplements for their product formulation and purity of ingredients through rigorous toxicology review.

NSF International created the NSF Certified for Sport program, which addresses the growing concerns of athletes and coaches about banned substances in supplements. This program focuses on minimizing the risk that a dietary supplement or ergogenic aid contains banned substances[49]—a tremendous safeguard for athletes, including tennis players. Look for the blue-and-white NSF safety stamp on dietary supplements.

ConsumerLab (CL) provides a third stamp of credibility. CL independently tests the quality of health and nutrition products, such as dietary supplements, publishing their test results and reviews found on their website, www.consumerlab.com. CL tests supplements for quality and safety. Their approval is designated by their blue-and-white logo on the packaging of supplements.

There are several organizations that provide credible information on dietary supplements for athletes. They include the National Center for Drug-Free Sport (www.drugfreesport.com), NSF International (www.NSFInternational.org), and the US Anti-Doping Agency (www.usada.org). These reliable resources can help tennis players make more selective choices about their dietary supplements.

Finally, researchers do not know the long-term effects of taking supplements over a period of time. This becomes a critical consideration during the childhood and teen years, when growth and development occur. Therefore, be selective about the supplements you put in your body, keeping in mind the following tips.

## BE A SAVVY SUPPLEMENTS CONSUMER

With the accessibility of supplements at your back door, from street-corner family drugstores to vitamin shops and Internet sites, be a savvy supplements consumer. Keep the following considerations in mind when purchasing supplements. These tips come from two sources: from the FDA's "Tips for Dietary Supplement Users: Making Informed Decisions and Evaluating Information," available on the FDA website,[50] and from the National Institutes of Health's Office of Dietary Supplements web page.[51]

1.  Supplements are designed to aid and abet the nutrition from our diet but not to replace the balance and variety of the foods we eat. Once again, effective tennis sports nutrition cannot happen by virtue of a supplement when proper nutrition is not at its base. Good diet first, supplements second, if necessary.

2.  Take a good look at your lifestyle. Ask yourself why you are taking a supplement. Could you get the same result by eating healthier foods? Or by managing stress? Could you feel more energetic by changing your sleep and exercise habits? Should you stop smoking or drink less? Working on improving your health behaviors is a much better investment than using a supplement as a quick fix for bad habits.

3.  Check with your doctor, pharmacist, or registered dietitian before using a supplement, particularly if you have such medical conditions as diabetes, hypertension, cancer, or heart disease. Supplements can contain strong active ingredients that could affect your body's systems, including breathing, circulation, and digestion.

4. Supplements may interact with prescription drugs and over-the-counter (OTC) medicines. Supplements contain active ingredients that can interact, even interfere, with the effectiveness of medication. For example, gingko biloba and vitamin E can thin the blood, as do aspirin and warfarin, a potent prescription blood thinner. Taking these supplements with these common OTC and prescription blood thinners could lead to excessive bleeding. High doses of gingko biloba can also decrease the effectiveness of antiseizure medication, such as Tegretol. Saint John's wort, an herbal supplement claiming to alleviate symptoms of depression, can reduce the effectiveness of prescription drugs for lowering cholesterol (statins) and for treating depression and seizures. Never underestimate the potential for drug-supplement or food-drug interactions; they can make a significant impact on your health.

5. After surgery, many people seek remedies to boost their nutrition and healing power. The FDA recommends refraining from taking supplements for at least two to three weeks after surgery to prevent potentially dangerous supplement and drug interactions that could affect healing, blood pressure, bleeding, and heart rate. Always consult with a doctor when starting a new supplement after surgery or medical procedures.

6. Children and teens should consult with their parents, coach, and health care professional before taking supplements. Because tennis players are driven to find ways to improve their athletic performance, they may seek the ergogenic potential of supplements. The lure is even stronger when supplements are directly marketed to youth and easily accessible for purchase. Parents need to stay alert and know what supplements their teens and children are using. Likewise, children and teens should

discuss their interest in taking a supplement with their parents and coach.

7. Be an informed consumer. Once again, the manufacturer is responsible for ensuring that supplements are safe and the claims on their labels are accurate before they are sold. If big dollars come before safety, consumers need to watch out. Keep in mind: the FDA is not responsible for testing the safety and effectiveness of supplements; this burden lies on the manufacturer who must comply with FDA's standards. Use critical thinking:

   a. Are the claims too good to be true? If a supplement claims to "cure" a disease or ailment or uses extreme descriptions, such as "miraculous results," "secret, ancient ingredient," or "never-discovered cure," be wary. Watch for strange terms that sound scientific and complex but have no meaning. Deciphering this language can be mystifying. Contact the manufacturer if you have questions. A simple phone call or e-mail should elicit an effective, accurate response from a responsible manufacturer. Seek out the expertise from a pharmacist or registered dietitian. If the manufacturer's goal is to aggressively sell its supplement with minimal regard for substantiating claims or considering safety, beware.

   b. Be careful not to fall in the testimonial trap. Anecdotes from self-proclaimed experts and testimonials from consumers (possibly make-believe ones, at that) can be highly influential in causing emotional decision making. The Internet, TV, blogs, Facebook posts, Twitter, and other social media can make these testimonials readily available to both adults and teens, who can misinterpret this as the truth when it can be fiction—the extreme opposite of the truth!

c. Report any adverse effects from the use of dietary supplements. Even if you are not sure the reaction was caused by the supplement, report it, whether you seek medical attention or not. The FDA contact number is 1-800-FDA-1088. Once reported, the FDA can keep track of complaints and research them. At the extreme, consumer safety complaints can get dangerous supplements off the market.

If you are considering taking a dietary supplement to improve your tennis performance, always consult with a professional first, such as a registered dietitian, pharmacist, or physician. Ergogenic aids are prevalent, but very few improve performance; they could even impede performance or, at worst, be unsafe and dangerous to use. Be aware that if supplements can't help, they can still hurt.

## CAN SUPPLEMENTS IMPROVE MY TENNIS GAME?

Knowing tennis players ambitiously seek ways to improve their game, resorting to ergogenic aids is common for both adults and children. In their position paper "Nutrition and the Athlete," the American College of Sports Medicine (ACSM) has classified ergogenic aids into four categories, based on the validity of their performance-enhancing claims:[52]

1. Ergogenic aids that perform as claimed
2. Ergogenic aids that may perform as claimed, but insufficient evidence exists on their claims
3. Ergogenic aids that do not perform as claimed
4. Ergogenic aids that are banned, illegal, or dangerous to use

Examples of dietary supplements in each category are discussed below.

**1. *Ergogenic Aids That Perform as Claimed.*** The ACSM lists several dietary supplements that have demonstrated strong enough evidence to sufficiently support their claim. However, minimal research has yet to be done on evaluating the impact of specific supplements on tennis performance. So, understand that these dietary supplements may or may not enhance your tennis performance.

**Creatine** is one of the most widely studied and used ergogenic aids. Creatine, a compound found in muscles, is an essential amino acid used in the body as a source of muscle energy. The ACSM deems creatine effective in repeated short bouts of high-intensity activity in sports that require bursts of energy from adenosine triphosphate, or ATP.[53] ATP is the fuel formed in our cells that is used for all energy-requiring processes, such as exercise. The energy produced by breakdown of ATP causes our muscles to contract: to bench press, to serve a tennis ball, to chase down a lob.

The body must constantly resynthesize or remake ATP. There is only a limited reserve of ATP to do a few seconds of exercise before needing to be resynthesized. Creatine may help reproduce ATP. Studies seem to support creatine's role. Creatine has been shown to increase body mass during weight training, although it is not as useful for endurance sports, like long-distance running.[54]

Based on creatine's ability to increase high-intensity exercise capacity, could it be a useful ergogenic aid in tennis, which requires the large muscles in our legs and arms to engage in continual stop-and-go bursts of energy? Pluim et al. examined tennis performance after a six-day creatine-loading phase and a four-week maintenance phase in one group of tennis players compared to a placebo group who did not receive creatine. Although the group given creatine did gain significant muscle mass (1.0–1.5

kg), there was no ergogenic benefit in tennis selective performance measures, such as serve and stroke velocity and sprint power.[55] Although sports science has not proven that creatine improves tennis performance, more studies need to be done. In fact, there is very limited literature on nutrition, dietary supplementation, and tennis performance.

Creatine supplementation is brought to life by the personal experiences from friend and tennis professional Tiffany Dabek Davis.[56] Davis had a successful professional career, highlighted by a qualifying spot in the 2005 US Open, beating international rising stars like Bulgaria's Tsvetana Pironkova along the way.

Davis also has the unique distinction of being a registered dietitian. Her nutrition knowledge gave her an edge. In her career, she strove to be the fittest player, beating many of her opponents through healthy diet and supplementation, including vitamins, whey protein, fish oil, and creatine.

Davis describes her personal experience with creatine monohydrate. She followed the loading phase of creatine supplementation in her off-season, working with Pat Etcheberry—arguably the world's best tennis fitness trainer, who has worked with countless pros, including Pete Sampras, Andre Agassi, Justine Henin, Martina Hingis, and Victoria Azarenka. Davis quickly gained five pounds of muscle in not much more than a week! Many athletes strive for this remarkable muscle metamorphosis. However, this gain in muscle mass actually hindered her professional game. Davis did not know how to use her newfound mass and strength. Eventually, she gave up on creatine and resorted to the healthy diet and selective supplement use that steered her to tennis success.

Creatine could be an option for grown adults who have developed good training habits and realize that there is no replacement for a healthy diet, exercise, and a conditioning program. Davis's experience with creatine supplementation exemplifies this. Teens and children should develop good habits in their diet and training program before resorting to creatine to enhance their tennis game. Young adults should also discuss the use of creatine with parents and coaches before taking it.

Although there is no agreement on the amount of creatine supplementation for ergogenic benefit, studies have demonstrated its efficacy with approximately a three-gram supplementation per day.[57] These studies use creatine monohydrate; many other forms of creatine are marketed to consumers, but most research is based on creatine monohydrate. Athletes usually take between three and five grams of creatine per day. Taking more of the suggested manufacturer dosing is rarely better. As with all supplements, follow the recommended dosage for creatine. The effects of decades of creatine use are unknown, since this supplement has only been available for about twenty years.

**Caffeine** is the most widely used and accessible ergogenic aid in the world. Caffeine is found naturally in coffee, tea, and cacao as well as esoteric plants such as the kola nut, guarana berries, and guayusa. Leaves of the guayusa tree are dried and brewed like a tea for their stimulative effects. The guarana plant produces fruit the size of a bean. Its seeds contain about twice the amount of caffeine in the same amount of coffee beans. Caffeine is added to sodas and energy drinks, many of which also contain naturally caffeinated guarana.

Caffeine is a central nervous system (CNS) stimulant. Since all sports, like tennis, require focus and alertness, athletes frequently use caffeine to enhance this aspect of their game. It is not surprising to see tennis players pull an energy drink or caffeinated soda from their tennis bags.

In addition to the stimulant effect of caffeine, research shows that caffeine improves physical endurance. Caffeine has been shown to enhance athletic performance in endurance sports, such as running, cycling, and cross-country skiing. Experts propose that caffeine increases muscle contractility, fat metabolism, and aerobic endurance.[58] Further study shows that caffeine may also be of benefit in high-intensity activities lasting up to twenty minutes, such as swimming and mid-distance running. This ergogenic effect can be achieved with as little as one hundred grams of caffeine, about the amount in eight ounces of brewed coffee.[59]

To study the effect of caffeine supplementation on tennis performance, researchers led by Damian Farrow at the Australian Institute of Sport evaluated caffeine use during prolonged simulated tennis matches. In this study, male elite tennis players were given three milligrams per kilogram of caffeine and then evaluated on specific measures of tennis performance, including stroke velocity, accuracy, and perceived exertion. The researchers found that caffeine supplementation increased serve velocity in the last set of the simulated match and diminished the effects of fatigue.[60]

As demonstrated by Farrow, the benefit of caffeine supplementation occurred with small to moderate levels of caffeine taken at a variety of times before, during, and end of activity. The men in the above study were given a dose of caffeine equivalent to about two to three eight-ounce cups of coffee at various times during tennis play. (Caffeine content of beverages and foods is listed in chapter 7).

Just because small to moderate amounts of caffeine may benefit your tennis game, large amounts of caffeine will not. Caffeine overload can cause anxiety, stomach distress, poor sleep, and heart palpitations. Since tennis relies so heavily on mental focus, caffeine-induced anxiety, jitteriness, and poor sleep will certainly deter performance.

In addition, caffeine-containing beverages like colas and tea should not be used for rapid hydration. A large cola or iced tea cannot replace fluids lost during exercise in the same way that water can. The body cannot keep up with caffeine metabolism when these drinks are rapidly consumed in large amounts. Caffeine can have a diuretic effect, making athletes lose water through frequent urination, also a deterrent to tennis performance. Water or sports drinks should be used for rehydration.

Since 2004, WADA has permitted caffeine as an ergogenic substance. However, caffeine is considered a "controlled and restricted substance" by the International Olympic Committee when an athlete reaches twelve micrograms per milliliter in a urine sample. Caffeine is on the restricted list by the NCAA when urine levels reach fifteen micrograms per milliliter in a sample.[61] A large amount of caffeine must be used before reaching this limit. In a typical male, this equates to five to six cups of coffee rapidly taken right before exercise—not a wise choice for most tennis players. Caffeine used in moderation and with discretion should be a safe ergogenic aid.

**Sports drinks** contain three necessary ingredients for athletic performance: water, carbohydrates, and electrolytes, including sodium and potassium. When used during extended exercise involving significant sweat loss, as occurs with tennis played in a hot climate, sports drinks are useful in replacing fluid and electrolytes lost in sweat. The carbohydrates or sugars in sports drinks replenish glucose stores needed by active muscles during tennis play. (Chapter 7 discusses the use of sports drinks in more detail.)

**Sodium bicarbonate.** When we do anaerobic exercise, like tennis, our blood becomes acidic from lactate or lactic acid buildup. Lactic acid is a normal by-product of anaerobic exercise. When stored carbohydrate in muscles is converted to energy or fuel in the absence of oxygen, lactic acid is produced. Although subject to debate, when too much lactic acid accumulates in the blood, early fatigue may result, impairing athletic performance.

Sodium bicarbonate, more familiarly known as baking soda, acts as a buffer to neutralize the acidity of the blood. Could this process delay fatigue in high-intensity exercise like tennis? Certainly, we all want our legs and forearms to be as spry at the end of a match as they are at the very beginning.

In a 2010 study, Ching-Lin Wu and his team studied the effect of bicarbonate supplementation on tennis performance. Researchers gave one group of tennis players bicarbonate supplementation and gave a placebo to the other group. The group of tennis players who received bicarbonate maintained their serves and ground strokes more consistently than the players who did not have the bicarbonate supplement. Wu found the difference in serve and ground stroke consistency to be significant.[62]

However, the potential side effects of taking sodium bicarbonate to relieve lactic acid "burn" could outweigh the benefits. Side effects of sodium bicarbonate supplementation initially occur in the digestive tract. They include gas, belching, nausea, and reflux. Unpleasant intestinal side effects include diarrhea and flatulence, undoubtedly obstacles on the tennis court.

Incidentally, lactic acid accumulation can be offset by proper training, warm down, adequate fluids, and a high-carbohydrate diet to ensure adequate glycogen stores.[63] These means of managing lactic acid buildup are far more beneficial than taking a bicarbonate supplement, especially if unpleasant gastrointestinal side effects develop on the court.

**Protein and amino acids.** Protein is comprised of amino acids, which help build and replenish muscle. Muscle is constantly getting worn and rebuilt in exercise. When protein intake is properly timed, it can enhance muscle repair and growth, improving the recovery process postexercise. The cycle of train, rest, and replete with protein is familiar to bodybuilders and other athletes.

Of note, protein supplements in their powder, liquid, or bar form have been found to be no more or less effective than supplementing with the same type and amount of protein found in food as long as adequate calories to build muscle mass are consumed.[64] These protein shakes, bars, and powders can also be high in refined sugars, fat, and calories.

Protein supplements serve their purpose in specific situations. When used in addition to high-quality protein in the diet, they provide a quick and convenient source for athletes on the go. If food sources are not readily available, protein bars, powders, and shakes are convenient and easy to use. Bars and most canned or bottled protein beverages are also nonperishable, whereas many food sources of protein are. This makes for easy travel in the backpack or tennis bag for busy tennis players. (Chapter 3 discusses protein in more detail.)

**2. Ergogenic Aids That May Perform as Claimed but Have Insufficient Evidence.** Some ergogenic aids have yet to produce enough evidence to definitively conclude that they do what they claim to do for the athlete. The ACSM includes glutamine, ribose, and beta-hydroxymethylbutyrate (HMB) in this category, to name a few.[65] The evidence is supportive at best. If enough evidence is produced, these supplements can move into category number one.

**3. Ergogenic Aids That Do Not Perform as Claimed.** This category contains the largest number of supplements. They have not demonstrated they perform as they claim. There is either no evidence or not enough to support that these supplements do what they claim to do; evidence may even support the opposite as research evolves. From taurine, oxygenated water, carnitine, and coenzyme Q10, these popular ergogenic aids sound good, but the ACSM states they have yet to produce evidence showing they do what they say they do to enhance athletic performance.[66]

Manufacturers must prove that their supplements perform as claimed. Studies to produce this kind of evidence can take time and cost money. The burden of producing conclusive evidence lies on the manufacturer, not the FDA. These supplements can move up the credibility rank if enough evidence is found to support their performance-enhancing claims.

**4. Ergogenic Aids That Are Illegal, Dangerous, or Banned.** All athletes should avoid this class of ergogenic aid. Without sufficient testing, adverse effects can occur—even death, as associated with ephedra supplementation and methylhexanamine, more familiarly known as DMAA. Ephedra contains ephedrine. Ephedrine promotes weight loss, but it also boosts heart rate and blood pressure, potentially causing heart attack, stroke, seizure, and even death. In 2004, the FDA banned ephedra. Thus far, ephedra has been the only dietary supplement banned by the FDA. You still see ephedra sold on websites and supplement shops. This is because it does not contain ephedrine but other extracts of the plant that are not likely to pose danger.[67]

Just because a supplement is not banned or misses the news for its notoriety, it does not mean it is safe. Consumers have reported hundreds of adverse reactions, many serious, including liver, kidney, and heart failure. A number of supplements are highly suspect for their safety, including colloidal silver and DMAA, a muscle-building, weight-loss supplement. In April 2013, the FDA deemed DMAA a dangerous, illegal dietary supplement after a number of deaths related to heart attack were associated with its use. DMAA is banned by WADA.

Like WADA, the International Tennis Federation (ITF) strives to maintain the integrity of tennis and to protect the health of tennis players participating in current events. ITF's nonapproved substance list mirrors WADA's. ITF prohibits the following abbreviated list of substances and methods in the tennis circuit, unless used for therapeutic reasons and within urine testing limits.[68] Refer to ITF's website for the comprehensive listing and tennis anti-doping education: www.itftennis.com/anti-doping.

# INTERNATIONAL TENNIS FEDERATION'S (ITF) ANTI-DOPING PROGRAMME LIST OF NONAPPROVED SUBSTANCES AND METHODS (2015)

## NONAPPROVED SUBSTANCES:

1. Anabolic agents, such as anabolic androgenic steroids
2. Peptide hormones, growth factors, related substances, and mimetics (e.g., erythropoietin, growth hormone, corticotrophins)
3. Beta-2 agonists
4. Hormone and metabolic modulators (e.g., insulin and estrogen receptor modulators, myostatin inhibitors)
5. Diuretics and other masking agents

## PROHIBITED METHODS:

1. Manipulation of blood and blood components (e.g., IV infusions or injections; administration of blood or red blood cells; any method used to artificially enhance uptake, transfer, or delivery of oxygen)
2. Chemical and physical manipulation (e.g., tampering or attempting to tamper with the validity of samples; IV infusions and injections of more than fifty milliliters per six-hour period, except those legitimately used in the course of medical care or clinical investigations)
3. Gene doping: use of normal or genetically modified cells

## PROHIBITED SUBSTANCES IN COMPETITION: TWELVE HOURS BEFORE SCHEDULED COMPETITION

1. Stimulants, such as amphetamine, adrenaline, phentermine
2. Narcotics (e.g., morphine, oxycodone, heroin)
3. Cannabinoids: natural (e.g., marijuana) or synthetic (e.g., 9-tetrahydrocannabinol, or THC)
4. Glucocorticosteroid—administered via oral, intramuscular, or rectal route

Competitive players governed under the rules of the ITF need to pay close heed to dietary supplement use, especially suspect ones that can be contaminated or impure. The ITF Anti-Doping Programme makes athletes responsible for any substances found in samples produced by them.

The ITF Anti-Doping Programme has an explicit warning about dietary supplements. They reiterate that some supplements may contain ingredients not listed on the label or in different quantities than stated on the label or even be contaminated with prohibited substances. These contaminants could be on the prohibited list, such as DMAA and testosterone. The consumption of a dietary supplement that contains a prohibited substance may subject a tennis player to penalties under the ITF Anti-Doping Programme. According to the ITF, a contaminated supplement will not excuse a positive doping test.[69]

As research progresses on dietary supplements and ergogenic aids, each study produces new and often conflicting results. This can be very confusing to the consumer. As studies become more sophisticated, we learn that what may have worked may end up not living up to its claim, and what was thought not to work may later be proven to be efficacious, even harmful. This is the nature of scientific research. Before a supplement's claim can be supported, there needs to be a consensus of replicated research. This produces the evidence that discerns fact from hype.

A good example of research gone full circle is the study of vitamin E's antioxidant impact. In the 1980s, leading experts unequivocally promoted vitamin E to be the heart-healthy vitamin. For quite some time, consumers self-prescribed vitamin E, religiously taking this supplement to ward off heart disease. However, evidence from most recent studies refutes theories about vitamin E and prevention of heart disease.

The Heart Outcomes Prevention Evaluation (HOPE) study, which followed 9,500 people with vascular disease or diabetes for 4.5 years, found those participants taking 400 IU of extra vitamin

E each day experienced no fewer and no more heart attacks than those without vitamin E supplementation. When many of these participants were followed for several more years, there was no significant protection vitamin E supplementation provided against heart attacks, strokes, and cancer. But there was a higher incidence of heart failure in the participants taking vitamin E.[70]

The National Cancer Institute (NCI) has reviewed nine randomized, controlled trials of dietary antioxidant supplementation on cancer prevention, one of which includes the HOPE study. The NCI summarizes that, to date, these trials do not provide enough evidence that dietary antioxidant supplements are beneficial in primary cancer prevention and that some trials even point to a higher rate of mortality with supplementation.[71] These studies used supplements and not food, a clear distinction, which supports the potential benefit of consuming these antioxidants from foods containing a mix of nutrition as opposed to the purified nutrient in supplement form.

One final note on nutritional supplements: they can be expensive—ridiculously expensive. When you add up the money spent on colorful bottles of supplements, as opposed to healthy foods containing the desired nutrient, you will appreciate the greater benefits of nutrition, taste, and satiety from eating whole foods. A whole-foods diet can cost a fraction of the same nutrition purchased through supplements with much more nutritional potency. Nutrients should come from whole foods first—then supplements, only when nutritional needs are not met with food.

## SHOULD I TAKE A SUPPLEMENT?

When it comes down to it, should tennis players take a supplement? Using a multivitamin supplement as "health insurance" to a good diet is a sound approach to ensure nutrient needs are met, while still striving for a diet rich in vegetables, fruits, whole grains, beans, legumes, lean protein, and low-fat dairy or dairy substitutes like soy.

Remember, good diet first, supplements second. A multivitamin that provides 100 percent of the Recommended Daily Allowance (RDA) for select nutrients is a safe approach when you make concerted efforts to meet your nutritional needs through diet first.

Consumers may have heard the term *Dietary Reference Intake* (DRI) and RDA used interchangeably. Deciphering the terminology can be confusing. What's the difference between a DRI and an RDA? The definitions are listed below.[72]

**Daily Reference Intake (DRI)**—the general collective term for reference values for nutrients used to plan and assess intakes of healthy people. These values include RDAs.

**Recommended Daily Allowance (RDA)**—the average daily level of intake sufficient to meet the nutrient requirements of nearly all healthy people.

**Adequate Intake (AI)**—an AI for a nutrient is only established if the RDA cannot be determined. A nutrient has either an RDA or an AI.

**Tolerable Upper Intake Level (UL)**—the highest daily intake of a nutrient that is likely to pose no risk of toxicity for almost all individuals.

**Estimated Average Requirement (EAR)**—the amount of nutrient that is estimated to meet the requirement of half of all healthy individuals in the population. EAR is not used for nutrient labeling, only RDA or AI.

Remember, the RDA covers nutrient requirements for practically all healthy people. Combining the nutrients from diet plus a multivitamin and mineral supplement (if needed) for 100 percent of the RDA will meet your micronutrient needs.

For those adhering to specific diets, individualize your supplementation based on those needs. If you know your diet is low in certain food groups, target that supplement. As an example, vegan diets, which restrict all animal products, can be low in vitamin B12, iron, zinc, and calcium (but rich in many nutrients from fruits, vegetables, and grains). These may be supplements of choice for someone on a vegan diet.

Certain conditions, such as celiac disease, Crohn's disease, and renal disease, necessitate dietary modifications, which may require supplements. Active tennis players with multiple food allergies or food intolerances may also be candidates for nutritional supplementation. A registered dietitian can help customize a supplement plan for tennis players based on their special dietary needs.

Be aware of the plethora of misleading information on ergogenic aids. Utilize those that have proven to do what they claim to do. Always let your coach, trainer, or parents know what supplements you are taking. Remember, all supplements contain active ingredients, so do your research on them, eat a good diet, and adopt healthy lifestyle behaviors before you seek to enhance your tennis game with supplements.

Let's revisit Andrea, who was introduced in the beginning of the chapter. Despite her good intent, she actually had too much control over her diet, her supplements, and her exercise habits, wreaking more havoc to her health than benefit. Andrea could even be exhibiting signs of orthorexia nervosa, an exaggerated concern with healthy eating so extreme that the obsession interferes with quality of life. Andrea sought nutritional counseling from a registered dietitian. With sound nutritional advice, combined with trust in her body's physiological signals for rest, Andrea was able to better manage her diet and supplement use—with better tennis stamina as a payoff.

# 3

# DEFYING PROTEIN
# PORTION DISTORTION

**The better I get, the more I realize how much better I can get.**
—Martina Navratilova

Sam is an eighteen-year-old elite athlete. He plays for both his nationally ranked high school baseball and tennis teams. At five foot nine, he competes with and against young men who are larger and more powerful. Most of his fellow baseball team players are over six feet tall, looming over his self-perceived modest physique. In order to gain muscle mass, Sam makes it a point to eat large amounts of protein—really large amounts. Sam's diet consists mostly of meat, refined carbs in bread and white rice, and about a half gallon of 2 percent milk each day. For insurance, he takes a whey protein shake after every gym workout. His diet provides about two hundred grams of protein per day. Sam feels that eating large amounts of protein will help him grow in the likeness of his formidable counterparts. Sam rarely eats fruits and vegetables. Like most active teens, fast food and soda are also staples in his diet. Sam gets sick a lot and finds this has taken its toll with his endurance on the tennis court and his long baseball practices. Could his diet be the reason?

Protein is one of three essential macronutrients in our diet. Macronutrients are required in large amounts and provide calories or energy. Carbohydrates and fat are the two other macronutrients. Protein is part of every cell tissue in our bodies. Protein provides amino acids necessary to build and repair muscle, cartilage, skin, and blood. Protein is also required to synthesize hormones and support the immune system, which helps fight infection and disease.

The amino acids in protein are the building blocks of muscle, skin, hair, and blood. There are twenty-one of these amino acids. Our bodies can make most of these amino acids, but eight of them, called essential amino acids, must come from protein in the foods we eat. In children, nine essential amino acids must come from food sources of protein.

The protein requirement for athletes is slightly higher than that recommended for nonathletes. However, many athletes, including tennis players, believe eating extra protein will boost muscle mass, power, and strength. They eat far too much protein, thinking that this extra protein converts to equivalent muscle mass. Believing that more steak means more muscle is a misconception. In the absence of the additional calories essential to build muscle, excess protein (30 percent or more of total calories) in a eucaloric (the calories needed to maintain the same body weight) diet does one of two things:

1. It is burned, or oxidized, as a fuel source—an expensive one at that.
2. It is stored as a fuel source called glycogen in muscles and liver for later use.

Furthermore, eating more protein and increasing total caloric intake without expending or burning these extra calories can lead to weight gain. These extra protein calories can be stored as fat, not muscle.

Yes, any calorie that is not utilized is stored, whether it is a calorie from carbohydrates, protein, or fat. This demonstrates our bodies' homeostatic drive to balance calories with energy expenditure. When enough calories are consumed to match those expended, weight maintenance occurs. When too few calories are consumed or too many expended to maintain weight, weight loss ensues. Finally, when more calories are consumed than the body needs and not enough are expended, this imbalance leads to overweight and obesity. (Chapter 6 discusses weight management in further detail.)

High protein intake does not correlate to equivalent muscle mass growth. Those extra protein calories that are used or stored as a fuel source are costly results of consuming too much protein in our diet—costly in that protein from animal sources tends to be far more expensive than protein from plant-based foods—and can be far less nutritious.

## HIGH-PROTEIN, LOW-CARB DIETS: NOT A TENNIS MATCH

High-protein, low-carb diets have become so mainstream, many regard them as conventional eating plans. Familiar high-protein, low-carb diets include the Atkins, Zone, Stillman, and Protein Power plans. Although these diets, like any reduced-calorie diet, provide a jump-start to weight loss, many people follow these diets for extended periods of time—months and even years.

Carbohydrates are the main fuel source for the brain, heart, kidneys, and skeletal muscle. Carbohydrates deliver the preferred fuel source to working muscles. They are critically important in fueling the working muscles. Restricting carbohydrates causes the body to go into a metabolic state called ketosis, whereby the body burns its own fat for fuel. Fuel or energy comes from ketones, the by-products made from the breakdown of fat stores.

Consuming too much protein, the equivalent of 30–50 percent or more of total caloric intake, coupled with too little carbohydrate, can have undesirable short- and long-term side effects. High-protein, low-carb diets can result in the following:[73]

1. *Undue stress on kidneys.* A high-protein diet stresses the kidneys and complicates preexisting kidney problems; results in high levels of protein in the urine; and can lead to kidney stones. Protein digestion produces waste products like urea. Kidneys need to work hard to flush urea and other waste products from our bodies. This places unnecessary stress on the kidneys.

2. *Ketosis.* As previously mentioned, ketosis occurs when the body burns its own fat stores for energy instead of glucose. This occurs in the absence of adequate carbohydrates, producing the waste by-product ketones. Contrary to how this sounds, burning fat for energy is not a physiologically normal process, compared to burning carbs for energy. In starvation, yes; for a healthy way to lose weight, no. Low-carb, high-protein diets restrict carbs in order to promote ketosis. Ketones can cause nausea, dizziness, decrease in appetite, and an uncanny fruity odor from the mouth, which can be socially undesirable. Ketosis can be prevented by the inclusion of at least one hundred grams of carbohydrate per day or the equivalent of four hundred calories from foods containing carbohydrates.

3. *Dehydration.* As kidneys filter and rid the body of the waste products from protein digestion, a significant amount of water is lost, leading to the risk of dehydration—not at all in the equation for tennis success. Initially, people may lose large amounts of weight on high-protein, low-carbohydrate diets, but much of this weight is total-body water loss.

4. *Satiety.* The feeling of fullness, which can be caused by eating too much protein, can suppress your appetite and cause you to not eat carbohydrates—the ideal fuel source for working muscles. The carbohydrates, fiber, vitamins, and phytonutrients in vegetables, fruits, and whole grains are valuable additions to the tennis player's diet that would otherwise be restricted on a high-protein, low-carbohydrate diet.

5. *Mobilize or leach calcium from the bones.* Acids are released by the body as protein is digested. These acids are buffered and absorbed with the help of calcium. The problem is that if you are not getting enough calcium from your diet, the body will mobilize or leach it from your bones, which can weaken them over time.

6. *Aggravate gout.* Gout is a condition characterized by excess uric acid accumulation, which causes swollen, red, and painful joints. Eating too much meat and seafood, both high-protein foods, may cause increased uric acid production, aggravating gout.

7. *Cause you to consume additional, unneeded saturated fat and cholesterol,* commonly found in foods high in animal protein. Fatty cuts of meat are high in saturated fat, which is the type of fat that raises blood cholesterol levels.

8. *Cause damage to your wallet and to the environment.* Foods high in animal protein are costly to not only your budget but also to the environment. Animal protein production demands significant resources, such as water, fuel, and labor, leaving a tremendous carbon footprint compared to the production of plant-based foods.

---

Producing just one pound of beef requires

- sixteen pounds of grain (which requires land, pesticides, water, fuel, and labor) and
- approximately 5,214 gallons of water (versus 23 gallons for one pound of tomatoes).

---

In fact, 70 percent of all grain produced in the world is consumed by livestock, not people. The Food and Agricultural Organization of the United Nations estimates livestock production generates nearly one-fifth of the world's greenhouse gases, more than both cars and planes.[74]

Does any nutrient or supplement, alone, build bulging muscle mass? The disheartening response, especially to the gym diehards, is "No." Resistance training and exercise, coupled with an increase in calories (approximately three hundred to five hundred per day) and an increase in protein, build muscle mass. This increase in protein can be met with the Western diet and, therefore, does not necessitate protein supplementation.[75]

Exercise causes the body to break down and resynthesize muscle tissue. Exercise (like tennis) causes the body to intentionally stress the muscle so that new muscle tissue is resynthesized. This wear and tear causes muscles to break down and rebuild.

Appropriately timed protein in an exercise program is also essential for proper recovery and immune function. Intense tennis conditioning and training put stress on the body, which can lower immune function. This makes athletes more susceptible to infections, like colds and other illness, as well as injuries. Protein provides high-quality amino acids to worn muscles for resynthesis and recovery.

## HOW MUCH PROTEIN IS ENOUGH?

The additional amount needed to serve this worthy purpose is much lower than most think. Factors influencing protein intake include protein quality, calorie and carbohydrate intake, type and intensity of exercise, and timing of protein intake.[76]

The RDA suggested by the American Academy of Sciences for sedentary, adult nonathletes is 0.8 grams of protein per kilogram of body weight or 0.36 grams per pound of body weight. Using this recommendation, a healthy 200-pound male would need about seventy-three grams of protein per day. A healthy 140-pound female would need fifty-one grams of protein per day.

Studies show athletes require a higher protein intake to help repair, resynthesize, and recover muscles from exercise and training. The American College of Sports Medicine (ACSM) suggests 1.2–1.4 grams per kilogram of body weight for endurance athletes, such as triathletes, cyclists, or marathon runners, and 1.2–1.7 grams per kilogram of body weight for strength-trained athletes or bodybuilders.[77]

The International Society of Sports Nutrition (ISSN) suggests 1.0–1.6 grams of protein for endurance athletes and 1.4–2.0 grams per kilogram of body weight for power- or strength-trained athletes. For competitive athletes engaged in intermittent sports, like tennis, the ISSN suggests an amount of protein in between this range, or approximately 1.4–1.7 grams per kilogram of body weight. These recommended amounts of protein, even at the higher end of the range, can be achieved by diet and should be safe in healthy, exercising adults.[78]

For competitive tennis players in the collegiate, semiprofessional, or professional circuit who engage in routine strength-training, conditioning, and/or endurance programs, the ISSN recommends a range of 1.4–2.0 grams per kilogram of body weight. The ISSN adds that this range applies to elderly athletes, as well.[79]

In his summary "Nutrition for Tennis: Practical Recommendations," Mayur K. Ranchordas, professor of sports and exercise nutrition suggests a protein level of 1.6 grams per kilogram of body weight for elite tennis players who undergo intense daily training.[80] This concurs with the ISSN recommendation. For a 150-pound athlete, this equals 109 grams of protein per day. Elite, competitive tennis players can achieve this amount in their diet without protein supplementation. Many young and elderly tennis players are probably meeting, if not exceeding, this protein allotment already.

Protein recommendation should be individualized, depending on duration and intensity of training. The harder the training day, lean more toward the upper limit of protein intake to support muscle repair and growth. On rest days or less-intense training days, the lower end of protein recommendation will suffice.

Remember, nutrient needs are dynamic and should adjust to your training needs accordingly.

Below is an example of how to calculate protein needs.

## Calculating Protein Needs

Tennis players can calculate protein needs using the following examples:

1. If your body weight is 150 lbs.:
   a. *Convert pounds to kilograms:*
      150 lbs. ÷ 2.2 lbs./kg = 68 kg
   b. *Multiply by the protein requirement:*
      68 kg × 0.8 g protein/kg = 54 g protein/day
      (RDA for sedentary nonathlete)
      68 kg × 1.4 g protein/kg = 95 g protein/day
      (endurance athlete)
      68 kg × 1.6 g protein/kg = 109 g protein/day
      (intermittent sports training, like soccer, tennis, football)
      68 kg × 2.0 g protein/kg = 136 g protein/day
      (strength/power training)

Most Americans, athlete or nonathlete, easily consume enough protein without even having to try! A three-ounce cooked portion of animal protein is the size and depth of a deck of playing cards. Three ounces of meat is equivalent to twenty-one grams of protein. An eight-ounce container of greek yogurt has eighteen grams of protein.

Protein is bountiful in our Western diet. Dine out at a typical American restaurant, and a ten-ounce steak or piece of salmon is common menu fare. This ten-ounce portion provides a whopping seventy grams of protein, more than the RDA for many Americans—on one dinner plate.

Combine these animal sources of high-quality protein with protein received from vegetables, grains, and dairy products, and the number adds up fast. Leave a deck of cards on your kitchen counter to keep you from protein-portion distortion. Remember, any excess calorie from protein (or fat or carbs) that is not needed could cause weight gain. Table 3.1 lists portion sizes and protein content from animal and plant foods.

**Table 3.1: Protein Content of Common Foods**

| Source | Portion Size | Protein (g) |
|---|---|---|
| **Animal:** | | |
| Chicken, white meat | 3 ounces | 21 |
| Chicken, dark meat | | |
| (medium leg and thigh) | 3 ounces | 21 |
| Beef, tenderloin | 3 ounces | 21 |
| Beef, lean hamburger | 3 ounces | 21 |
| Beef, ground chuck | 3 ounces | 21 |
| Fish, white (cod, tilapia) | 3 ounces | 21 |
| Fish, coldwater (salmon) | 3 ounces | 21 |
| Tuna, albacore, in water | 3 ounces | 21 |
| Eggs | 1 large | 7 |
| Yogurt (1% milk fat) | 8 ounces | 10 |
| Greek yogurt | 8 ounces | 18 |
| Cheese (Cheddar) | 2 ounces | 14 |
| **Plant:** | | |
| Veggie burger | 1 2.5-ounce patty | 11 |
| Tofu | 4 ounces | 10 |
| Nut butter (peanut, almond) | 3 tablespoons | 9 |
| Almonds | 1/4 cup | 5 |
| Beans (soy, garbanzo) | 1 cup, cooked | 14 |
| Legumes (lentils) | 1 cup, cooked | 14 |
| Quinoa | 1 cup, cooked | 24 |
| Edamame | 1/2 cup | 9 |

Tennis players need to match protein intake with type and intensity of exercise. Competitive tennis players tend to be less bulky, unlike their football player counterparts, who may be twice the size and weight. Strength-trained athletes like football players and weight lifters generally have higher protein needs than tennis players.

As tennis legend Nick Bollettieri says of Roger Federer's fluid, graceful movement on the court: "He moves without moving."[81] Without doubt, Roger Federer's amazing success is a result of his outstanding physical conditioning adapted to his tennis goals. Federer's tennis fitness, combined with his on-court acumen, results in impeccable footwork and movement efficiency. No doubt, tennis aficionados deem him the greatest player of all time—his success credited to his magical movement and perfect positioning on the court.

Tennis play requires many facets of athletic performance: quickness, flexibility, strength, movement efficiency, balance, cardiovascular fitness, and endurance, generally supported by a leaner body build. Certified athletic trainers provide tennis-specific conditioning to train the body for the demands of tennis.

Diet should be no different. A dietary regimen should also match training goals. Sporting excess muscle mass through "bulking up," errantly consuming copious amounts of protein and calories, may actually impede the requisite bursts of quick and agile movements required for top tennis performance.

It is easy to get caught up in the hype of misinformation about protein, especially at the gym, at vitamin/supplement stores, and through television and the Internet. Aside from the common goal of winning, different athletes have different physical fitness and dietary protein targets.

Clearly, our challenge lies not in achieving enough protein but in managing protein overload. Americans are fortunate to have an abundant food supply. Dana Gunders reports through the Natural Resources Defense Council that up to 40 percent of all food produced in the United States is discarded—and that is before it even gets to the table.[82] In American homes across the country, plates are brimming with food, including animal protein.

Typical homemade meals in your own kitchen can exceed reasonable protein portion sizes. Order a meal from an American restaurant, and you will be served two to even three times more animal protein than you require. This portion distortion could easily equate to the full day's allowance of protein in one sixteen-ounce rib-eye steak.

Portion distortion is brainwashing the public into thinking large protein portion sizes are the norm while providing way more calories, saturated fat, and cholesterol than needed. Again, any extra calorie that is not utilized for energy is either stored as glycogen for fuel or converted to excess body weight, which leads to overweight and obesity.

## PROTEIN AND NUTRITION FOR THE VEGETARIAN TENNIS PLAYER

Vegetarian diets have become the diet of choice for many athletes, including tennis players. Vegetarian diets have clear health benefits. Good vegetarian diets are high in fiber and antioxidants and low in saturated fat and dietary cholesterol. I know several vegetarian tennis players who are able to balance good nutrition with their active tennis lifestyles.

There are several different types of vegetarian diets. Vegan diets, which eliminate all animal sources, including dairy and eggs, rely solely on plant-based foods for protein and nutrients. Lacto-ovo vegetarian diets—which eliminate meat, poultry, and fish but include eggs and dairy products—can more readily meet iron, protein, and calcium needs. Flexitarian or semivegetarian diets are primarily plant based but do include small amounts of animal protein. Flexitarians or "flexible vegetarians" go meatless most of the time but do not completely give it up. Those who say they are vegetarian and eat small amounts of chicken, beef, or fish are semivegetarians or flexitarians.

Tennis players choosing a vegan diet need to be diligent about getting the nutrients they need for tennis performance. Carefully planned vegan diets can meet all nutritional needs for athletes. There are many athletes who have adapted a vegan lifestyle. Several notable vegan athletes include the following:

- Carl Lewis, track-and-field Olympian
- Desmond Howard, Heisman Trophy winner, former Green Bay Packer, and ESPN analyst
- Rich Roll, American triathlete
- Mike Tyson, former heavyweight boxer
- Ricky Williams, Heisman Trophy winner and former Miami Dolphins running back
- Tony Gonzalez, former Atlanta Falcons football player
- Venus Williams, tennis superstar

Although Martina Navratilova recently started eating an occasional fish meal, she is, without doubt, tennis's most acclaimed vegetarian.

When vegan diets are not well planned, they can be inadequate, even deficient in key nutrients—including protein, iron, zinc, vitamin B12, creatine, and calcium. These nutrient deficiencies can affect tennis performance.

**Protein.** Although protein needs should be sufficiently met in a vegan diet through vegetables, grains, beans, peas, nuts, and soy, special considerations for protein requirements need to be made for vegan tennis players, who get their protein exclusively from these plant sources. Because amino acids in plant-based foods are less bioavailable than those obtained through animal sources, vegan athletes should add 10 percent to the protein requirements listed above. Bioavailability is the rate at which the body is able to absorb nutrients. As an example, a sixty-gram protein requirement for a nonvegan becomes a sixty-six-gram protein requirement for a vegan athlete.

The biological value of protein influences its bioavailability. Biological value measures the protein quality—ultimately, how much of the nitrogen in their amino acids is used for tissue formation divided by the nitrogen absorbed from the food source. This number is multiplied by 100 to get an index or biological value rating. The biological value measures how efficiently the body uses the protein consumed in the diet.

Animal protein typically has a higher biological value (HBV) than vegetable sources of protein. Eggs and whey protein have a biological value of 100, meaning that all the nitrogen in their amino acids is used by the body. Formerly known as a *complete* protein, protein sources that contain all essential amino acids, like eggs, are termed *high-quality* protein sources. By definition, since most plant-based protein sources do not contain all eight essential amino acids, they do not provide high-quality protein. The exception is the high-quality protein in vegetable sources such as soy, spirulina, and quinoa.

By no means is the protein in plant-based diets inferior to that of animal-based diets. Beans are excellent sources of protein but lack the amino acid methionine. Grains lack the essential amino acid lysine but contain methionine. If both of these foods are eaten, there is no need to worry about getting high-quality protein. Their limiting amino acids complement each other. And no longer do vegans need to complement protein sources (e.g., beans and rice) in one sitting by eating them in the same meal. As long as a variety of vegetable sources are consumed throughout the day—from grains, vegetables, seeds, nuts, beans, and legumes—a vegan will receive a good variety of complementary amino acids to fulfill protein need.

Biological value does not take into account key factors that influence the digestion of protein, such as preparation and cooking. Biological value also does not factor in the interaction of other foods before absorption, which is more closely related to the concept of bioavailability. Nutrients in vegetable sources of protein tend to be less bioavailable than nutrients in animal sources of protein.

**Vitamin B12** has many functions, including the synthesis of red blood cells, which carry oxygen throughout our bodies. Even though vitamin B12 is made by microorganisms in our large intestines, we still require an outside source from foods to ensure that our needs are met. Vitamin B12 is abundant in meat, poultry, eggs, and other animal foods, as compared to plant-based foods. The vegan tennis player should take a vitamin B12 supplement to meet the RDA of 2.4 micrograms of vitamin B12 per day.

**Iron** is a component of hemoglobin, the protein in our red blood cells that carries oxygen from our lungs to our working muscles. The oxygen is needed to oxidize, or burn, carbohydrates for energy. Hemoglobin also carries the important molecule nitric oxide. The RDA for iron is eight milligrams for men and eighteen milligrams for women—until menopause, after which it goes back to eight milligrams.

Iron depletion, the first stage of iron deficiency, is the most common iron deficiency seen in male and female athletes. Iron depletion is much more prevalent in women. Research shows that 9–12 percent of non-Hispanic white women in the United States can be iron deficient. The incidence is higher in African American and Mexican American women, at 20 percent.[83] Symptoms of iron depletion include fatigue, dizziness, headaches, and weakness—obvious adversaries on the tennis court.

Maintaining adequate iron intake can be challenging for teenage girls and adult female tennis players due to losses through menstruation. Combined with a low iron intake from a vegan or calorie-restricted diet, iron depletion occurs. Causes of iron depletion include the following:

- low dietary intake of iron
- low bioavailability of dietary iron
- body losses—through menstrual loss or excessive loss in heavy sweating
- destruction of red blood cells or hemolysis—the stress of running in tennis and other sports that involve significant pounding impact can destroy red blood cells[84]

Serum ferritin is a measure of iron levels in your blood. Ferritin is the body's storage form of iron. Normal ferritin levels are 12–300 ng/dl for men and 12–150 ng/dl for women. Your physician can evaluate your ferritin levels.

If you are iron deficient, you may need to increase your dietary iron intake or even take an iron supplement. Always take iron supplements under the guidance of your doctor. Your doctor will prescribe the proper amount of iron to ensure you are not getting too much or too little. Because iron therapy can be prolonged, a few days of iron supplementation will not be enough to restore your iron to normal levels. It takes about four months to restore iron stores to normal levels.

Replenishing iron through diet can be challenging for vegan tennis players. There are two types of dietary iron: heme and nonheme iron. Heme iron is found in animal products like beef, poultry, pork, and eggs. Nonheme iron is found in plant-based foods such as spinach, beans, raisins, and iron-fortified cereals. The body absorbs heme iron much better than nonheme iron.

Tips for vegans to enhance iron intake and absorption:

- Select iron-enriched and iron-fortified breads and cereals. Keep in mind that many of these fortified foods may have a high iron content on the label, but the amount of this nonheme iron that is absorbed is significantly lower—only about 10 percent absorption.

- Eat iron-fortified foods with vitamin C. Vitamin C enhances the absorption of nonheme (and heme) iron. Have iron-fortified breakfast cereal with a glass of vitamin C–rich orange or grapefruit juice.
- Use a cast-iron skillet for cooking. Traces of iron can end up in the food cooked in it, increasing the iron content of that food.
- Avoid drinking coffee, wine, or tea with meals—coffee, wine, and tea contain substances called tannins that can decrease the absorption of a number of minerals, including iron. Drink your coffee before you eat your meal rather than afterward to improve iron absorption.

**Zinc** is a mineral needed by about one hundred enzymes in our bodies that carry out essential processes. Zinc also plays a role in immune function, wound healing, and protein synthesis. This is the RDA for zinc:

| Age | Males | Females |
| --- | --- | --- |
| 9–13 years | 8 mg | 8 mg |
| 14–18 years | 11 mg | 9 mg |
| 19+ years | 11 mg | 8 mg |

Grains, legumes, nuts, tofu, and oatmeal are sources of zinc in the vegan diet. Although vegans should not have a difficult time getting enough zinc in the diet, like iron, the zinc in plant-based foods is much less absorbable than the zinc found in beef. Many of these plant-based foods—including grains, legumes, and nuts—contain phytates, substances that decrease the absorption of several minerals, including iron, zinc, and calcium. It is suggested that vegans may require as much as 50 percent more zinc than nonvegetarians.[85]

Ways vegans can enhance the bioavailability of zinc include the following:

- Soak beans, grains, and seeds in water several hours before cooking.
- Consume more leavened grain products, such as bread, compared to unleavened grains (e.g., crackers). The leavening process partially breaks down the phytates in grains that limit the absorption of nutrients.[86]

If you are considering going vegan, consult with a registered dietitian beforehand to ensure your nutrient needs are met. Meeting nutrient needs is the foundation for tennis performance—with animal protein or without.

## GLUTEN-FREE: IS IT THE TENNIS PLAYER'S DIET?

Many of today's tennis stars attribute the gluten-free diet to their meteoric tennis success. Novak Djokovic, Andy Murray, Sabine Lisicki, and Bethanie Mattek-Sands credit their tennis success, in great part, to the gluten-free diet. What is the tennis world's affinity for the gluten-free diet?

Djokovic has most notably brought the gluten-free diet to tennis, stunning the world with his incredible tennis run in 2011 shortly after realizing he was gluten sensitive. So convinced by his gluten-free makeover, Djokovic credits his diet and lifestyle changes in his 2013 personal story *Serve to Win: The 14-Day Gluten Free Plan for Physical and Mental Excellence*.

In Hannah Britt's September 10, 2013, news feature for the United Kingdom's *Daily Express*, Djokovic admits struggling with asthma-like symptoms, fatigue, and lack of focus during his most high-profile matches, including the Grand Slams. Thinking it would keep up his energy level, he states he ate bread, pasta, and pizza from his parents' restaurant and candy bars and sugary foods during his matches. After a travesty of a loss in the 2010 quarterfinals of the Australian Open against Jo-Wilfried Tsonga, Djokovic drastically changed his diet. With nutritional guidance, Djokovic eliminated gluten and focused on a healthy diet, and the rest of 2011 becomes tennis history: ten titles (including three Grand Slams), a forty-three-match winning streak, and the fulfilled dream of becoming the number-one male tennis player in 2011. Djokovic's success continues, still number one in the world as of 2015.

Djokovic's well-publicized gluten-free diet may make you want to jump on the gluten-free bandwagon yourself. Tennis superstar Andy Murray did, as well as Sabine Lisicki. If only a fraction of our tennis game could follow in the footsteps of Djokovic's (or Murray's or Lisicki's) accomplishments, most of us would find this diet very enticing. However, a gluten-free diet, like any diet, needs to be explored for the right reasons.

You may wonder why a discussion of the gluten-free diet comes in a chapter on protein. Although commonly found in foods high in carbohydrates, like bread and pasta made from wheat, gluten is actually a protein. More technically, gluten is the collective term for the amino acid sequences found in wheat, barley, rye, and oats. Many foods—such as fruits, vegetables, eggs, meat, poultry, fish, and certain grains and starches—are gluten-free, making it fairly easy to obtain variety and good nutrition on a gluten-free diet.

**Table 3.2: Starches and Grains Allowed and Restricted on a Gluten-Free Diet**

| Allowed | Restricted |
|---|---|
| Rice (brown and white) | Barley |
| Corn and Cornmeal | Bulgur |
| Quinoa | Couscous |
| Teff | Dinkel/Spelt |
| Millet | Durum |
| Arrowroot | Einkorn wheat (Triticum) |
| Amaranth | Emmer wheat (Farro) |
| Flax | Graham Flour |
| Soy | Kamut (Khorasan wheat) |
| Sorghum | Matzo meal |
| Tapioca | Malt (extract, flavoring, syrup, vinegar) |
| Buckwheat | Orzo |
| Hominy | Rye |
| Yucca | Oats (most commercial) |
| Nut flour | Wheat (bran, germ, starch, cracked wheat) |
| Oats (uncontaminated) | |

Two conditions warrant the need for a gluten-free diet: celiac disease and the more ambiguous gluten sensitivity. Celiac disease, or celiac sprue, is an autoimmune disorder and inherited intolerance to gluten. In celiac disease, gluten is resistant to digestion. When consumed, it causes the immune system to produce antibodies, which attack the small intestine. The small intestine has fingerlike projections, called villi, which absorb nutrients entering the bloodstream. When the immune system detects gluten and turns against the body, it attacks the villi of the small intestine, preventing nutrients from being absorbed. Malabsorption occurs. Symptoms include abdominal pain, diarrhea, and weight loss. Celiac disease is diagnosed by blood tests, genetic testing, and biopsy of the small intestine. The only treatment for celiac disease is lifelong adherence to a gluten-free diet.

Celiac disease is not the same as a wheat allergy. An allergy is an immune response to food. The body treats the food item or allergen as a foreign, harmful substance and attacks it. This reaction by our immune system produces many symptoms, such as swelling of the lips, face, throat, and tongue; diarrhea; shortness of breath; and anaphylaxis, a very severe, life-threatening allergic reaction. An allergist should diagnose a food allergy using proven diagnostic methods, such as skin-prick test, blood test, oral food challenge, or elimination diet. Children commonly have food allergies but may grow out of them as they get older, whereas adults do not.

Adults can confuse gluten allergy with nonceliac gluten sensitivity—very different terminology. Nonceliac gluten sensitivity is a more nebulous condition than celiac disease or wheat allergy. People who have celiac disease–like symptoms, such as bloating, diarrhea, cramps, and headaches, seem to find relief by eliminating gluten, although they are not diagnosed with celiac disease or wheat allergy. They do not experience the physiological damage to the small intestine like those with celiac disease. Those who are gluten sensitive may tolerate very small amounts of gluten, whereas people with celiac disease may not be able to tolerate even the smallest trace of gluten in a bread crumb!

Currently, there is no gold-standard testing to diagnose gluten sensitivity. Many experts suggest using an elimination diet in which gluten-containing foods are avoided for a period of time to determine if symptoms abate. The parallel option to an elimination diet is a "challenge," whereby gluten-containing foods are given in small increments. You and your health professional evaluate symptoms to determine what amount of gluten is tolerable.

*Blood testing for gluten sensitivity.* Blood tests for food sensitivities and intolerances have become popular. Most blood tests measure the immune response to over 350 antigens in various foods, including gluten. Antigens are substances in food (and in the envi ronment) that cause the white blood cells in our immune system to produce antibodies against it. Our bodies produce their own antibodies when they identify foreign substances (antigens) and then go to work to neutralize them. Your own body also forms antigens such as toxins. If you have a sensitivity to the food antigen, your body will treat it as if it were a foreign substance. In the blood test, you send a sample of your blood to the lab where reaction to different food antigens can be tested.

Be wary of these blood tests for the following reasons. These tests may produce variations depending on immune response, stress level, and illness on the given day your blood is drawn. These blood tests can tell you to avoid a long list of many of your favorite healthy foods, like fresh vegetables, fruits, soy, and grains, which you may only have a mild sensitivity to (or not). Your immune response to these foods may be so benign you do not experience any symptoms of a sensitivity at all. By eliminating a laundry list of healthy foods, you may be doing your body more harm than good. It is important to know that these blood tests do not diagnose food allergies. An allergy test evaluates the allergy-type antibodies released in the bloodstream known as immunoglobulin E (IgE) antibodies. Allergies provoke a different immune response compared to a food sensitivity's response. Finally, these blood tests can be expensive.

You have lived with your body all your life and know it the best. Use common sense when evaluating these blood tests for food sensitivity. If you are uncertain how to evaluate these tests, seek assistance from a knowledgeable health professional.

Undeniably, people have nonceliac gluten sensitivity—but who they are and how many is unclear. Many of the symptoms related to gluten sensitivity could be the result of an array of nutrient deficiencies. There is a wide range of reported symptoms, including abdominal pain, constipation alternating with diarrhea, loss of appetite, depression, anxiety, headache, chronic fatigue, reflux, insomnia, and eczema. Experts suggest people with celiac disease–like symptoms try an exclusion of gluten for three months to determine if symptoms are the result of gluten sensitivity.[87]

From celebrities to athletes who follow a gluten-free diet, one would think this is just another diet trend. Yet, this is not true. Celiac disease and gluten sensitivity are on the rise, particularly in younger folks. Celiac disease, once thought to occur in one in every three hundred Americans, has increased to one in every one hundred Americans.[88] Easier and more accurate diagnosis of the disease has likely affected the increase in these numbers. Still, only about 10 percent of those are diagnosed. Confusing the symptoms of celiac disease or gluten sensitivity with other gastrointestinal conditions, such as colitis or irritable bowel syndrome, is one reason for this underdiagnosis.

Another popular yet unproven theory is that the increase in celiac disease could be in the wheat itself. Over the decades of food industrialization, processed foods containing wheat have a higher gluten content. Additionally, crossbreeding of wheat to make it hardier and more abundant may have caused consumers to have a greater sensitivity to its gluten content or composition— becoming less tolerant of wheat's genetic modification.

Like celiac disease, treatment of gluten sensitivity is a strict gluten-free diet. Common foods restricted include foods made with wheat, including bread, pasta, cereals, and baked goods, as well as oats, barley, and rye. Foods permitted include potato, rice, corn, quinoa, wheat berry, and soy. Tennis players with gluten sensitivity need to ensure their diets have adequate energy-producing carbohydrates to make up for foods that are eliminated in a gluten-free diet. Make sure you have the proper gluten-free nutrition for tennis play by seeking nutritional advice from a registered dietitian.

When does gluten-free become fad versus fact? When people resort to gluten-free diets for weight loss or as a panacea for their gastrointestinal or many other health concerns for no diagnosed reason, then the gluten-free fad overtakes reason. I know many people who have gone gluten-free; when I ask them why, they have no idea other than "everyone else is doing it"—not the right reason to be on a gluten-free diet.

Gluten-free diets are not weight-loss diets. When people eliminate gluten from foods like bread and pasta and do not replace those calories with other foods, they will lose weight. Reducing calories causes the weight loss, not reducing gluten. Many tennis players have proudly told me they have lost weight on a gluten-free diet, not realizing that it was due to a calorie reduction, not a gluten reduction.

When consumers preemptively resort to a gluten-free diet to address their gastrointestinal, weight, or other medical problems, they may not seek the professional attention they really need to diagnose and treat their true condition. Similar gastrointestinal symptoms may be related to irritable bowel syndrome, diverticulosis, food allergies, Crohn's disease, colitis, or leaky gut syndrome, all of which require medical attention. They also exclude the fiber, vitamins, and phytonutrients from healthy foods, such as whole-grain bread, pasta, and cereal, spending time and energy purchasing gluten-free foods when they are not needed.

Thankfully, sifting through shelves of gluten-free food products in the market has become easier with the FDA's gluten-free ruling. Effective August 5, 2014, this ruling provides guidelines manufacturers must follow to label their foods *gluten-free*. It also creates standardization of what *gluten-free* exactly means, thereby protecting consumers from misleading marketing. If you decide you want to make the gluten-free move, seek advice from your doctor and registered dietitian for gluten-free guidance.

## Pre- and Post-Tennis Protein Timing

A good sports nutrition program provides adequate nutrients coupled with their timing for peak athletic performance. Protein serves its purpose in tennis when it is appropriately timed before and after match play. Studies strongly support the role of protein timing in athletic performance and recovery.[89]

Small amounts of protein, along with carbohydrates approximately three to four hours before exercise, provide satiety to satisfy hunger, helps build and repair muscle tissue, and may help reduce postexercise muscle soreness. Eating protein early enough will also ensure that your body has time to digest it before you walk on court. Post-tennis protein repairs and resynthesizes worn muscle. Protein consumed after exercise also enhances glycogen synthesis, especially important in tournament play when adequate fuel is required for a subsequent match.

Planning nutrition the day of a tennis match (and well-before that) ensures that you will have the proper balance of fuel to take on tennis's unpredictable demands for endurance, energy, and mental focus. The below pre- and post-tennis nutrition plan is also outlined in chapter 10 for easy reference.

## THREE TO FOUR HOURS BEFORE TENNIS— CHOOSE A LIGHT MEAL

- eight ounces of greek yogurt and a half cup of fresh fruit topped with a quarter cup of cereal or granola
- peanut butter and all-fruit jam on toast and eight ounces of chocolate milk
- turkey, tuna, or lean roast-beef sandwich and piece of fruit
- lean hamburger or veggie burger on a whole-wheat bun with lettuce and tomato and baked chips
- bagel sandwich with egg and piece of fruit
- sports bar and twelve-ounce fruit smoothie

# THIRTY TO SIXTY MINUTES BEFORE TENNIS

Foods eaten thirty to sixty minutes before exercise should be easy-to-digest carbohydrates rather than protein. Consuming carbohydrates right before a match also ensures that blood glucose levels are sustained for quick energy. Consume about fifteen to thirty grams of carbohydrates shortly before your match. Examples of easy-to-digest carbohydrates include the following:

- crackers, pretzels, baked chips
- a piece of fruit: medium banana or medium apple, peach, pear
- sports beans and gels (amount equivalent to fifteen to thirty grams on label) or eight ounces of sports drink
- granola or cereal bar

By all means, do not eat a large protein and fat-laden meal right before a tennis match. At many tennis tournaments, hot dogs, hamburgers, nachos, pizza, fries, and soda are common fare for between-match foods that hungry children and teen tennis players gravitate toward. The intention to select salads is good, but when they are laden with several ounces of high-fat Caesar or ranch dressing, they are also not a good choice.

The availability of these high-fat foods, combined with hearty, ravenous appetites can cause children, teens, and grown-ups to consume a high-fat, high-protein meal prior to their next match. These high-protein, high-fat foods can result in exercise-induced indigestion on the court, characterized by bloating, cramping, gas, flatulence, and nausea.

Protein and fat take several hours to digest, compared to carbohydrates. Limit protein and fat right before a tennis match. They take longer to digest than carbohydrates, making you feel full and even sluggish when you walk on the court. Your body needs to focus on exercise—and not on digestion—before your big match.

# AFTER-TENNIS NUTRITION

After your tennis "workout," match, or vigorous exercise of at least twenty minutes or more, muscles are primed and ready to accept carbohydrates and protein to nourish, repair, and build new muscle, as well as to restore glycogen, the storage form of carbohydrate. Tennis, like most athletics, results in normal microtrauma to muscles and joints. Protein, carbohydrates, and good nutrition repair and rebuild this worn muscle and boost the immune system. This postexercise window, approximately forty-five minutes long, is a golden opportunity to replenish these thirsty muscles for efficient exercise recovery.

Consume these ideal post-tennis workout foods containing protein and carbohydrates within forty-five minutes after your tennis match:

**Table 3.3: Carbohydrate and Protein Content of Post-Tennis Workout Foods**

| Food Item | Carbohydrate (g) | Protein (g) |
|---|---|---|
| 16 oz. chocolate milk | 35 | 16 |
| 1 turkey sandwich on whole-grain bread with 2 oz. turkey, light mayo, mustard, tomato | 35 | 20 |
| 1 cup whole-grain dry cereal, banana, 8 oz. soy or skim milk | 47 | 14 |
| Smoothie: 8 oz. yogurt, 1 cup fresh fruit, 1/2 cup skim or soy milk | 45 | 12 |
| 8 oz. of greek yogurt and one medium banana | 30 | 20 |

Even though protein needs can be met through diet, many athletes, including tennis players, seek protein supplements via powders, drinks, and elixirs. Indeed, protein is one of the most in-demand nutrients that adorn supplement shelves. Protein supplements are convenient and easy to use when dietary sources are not readily available.

Whey protein has received the most attention as the postexercise protein supplement of choice for a reason. Whey protein contains branched-chain amino acids (BCAAs). Leucine, isoleucine, and valine are BCAAs. BCAAs bypass the liver and absorb directly into the bloodstream, where muscles can utilize them quickly and efficiently to repair and build new tissue. BCAAs are in animal protein in the proper ratio. Foods like yogurt, milk, and lean meat, chicken, fish, and poultry supply BCAAs.

Although protein supplements are convenient, they cannot replace the high-quality protein (and taste) found in whole foods. Utilizing whole foods can simply be done by replacing a protein supplement with a turkey sandwich or low-fat chocolate milk. Both of these foods contain carbohydrates to replenish muscle glycogen stores and all essential amino acids, including BCAAs, to nourish, repair, and build muscle. Food sources of nutrients (versus supplements) provide additional nutrition, fiber, vitamins, minerals, and phytonutrients—many of which researchers are still finding to be beneficial to our health.

There are components in food that cause protein and other nutrients to be more bioavailable—that is, digested, absorbed, and utilized better by the body. In most cases, food sources of protein can be less expensive than supplements. Make every attempt to get your nutrients, including protein, from food sources. The ISSN's position on protein supports using foods first.[90] When that is not possible, a protein supplement or drink, particularly during the postworkout window, is effective for muscle synthesis and recovery.

The two key takeaways on protein nutrition:

1. Incorporate the proper amount of protein in your tennis diet. Consume enough calories and protein to nourish, build, and repair muscles, while avoiding protein portion distortion.
2. Timing of nutrients is important. Time protein intake around tennis match play, pre- and post-tennis, to optimize its ergogenic effect.

Chapter 10 provides further suggestions for protein and carbohydrate intake before, during, and after various tennis scenarios for optimal performance and recovery.

Remember Sam, who was introduced in this chapter? He had been mistakenly consuming too much protein from high-fat, high-calorie food sources while eating too little of any other nutritious foods, including fresh fruits, vegetables, and whole grains. Thinking the protein in his food equated to bulging muscles, Sam filled up on high-fat meat, milk, and protein supplements. He excluded essential vitamins, minerals, phytonutrients, and fiber from fruits, vegetables, and whole grains needed to keep him healthy.

After seeking nutritional guidance, he tapered his protein intake to his baseball and tennis training regimen. He enhanced his nutrition with immune-building phytonutrients from the vegetables, fruits, and whole grains he liked to eat. He accepted his size and weight status. He became leaner, increasing his agility and speed on both the tennis court and baseball field. He felt better, got sick less often, and improved his overall health. He reaped the quintessential reward from his diet makeover by helping his baseball team win its elite high school district title.

# 4

## DOES FAT MAKE YOU FAT?

**If you can react the same way to winning and losing, that's a big accomplishment … Quality is important because it stays with you the rest of your life.**
—Chris Evert

Marsha has been struggling to lose weight for years. As a fifty-four-year-old club doubles player, Marsha feels she can reach the next USTA level if she loses those stubborn extra twenty pounds. This would clearly improve her fitness on the court. Marsha has desperately tried diet after diet, resorting to infomercials, WebMD, and *The Dr. Oz Show* as her resources. Over the years, she has spent thousands of dollars on dehydrated and frozen meals, diet plans, and exercise gadgets. Marsha decided she would simply keep her fat intake to fewer than thirty grams per day. She vigilantly read labels. She logged fat grams. Despite her enthusiasm about an initial three-pound drop in weight, mostly from water and muscle loss, Marsha's weight plateaued. Marsha's cravings for food—particularly bread, pasta, and sweets—were uncontrollable. Perplexed, cranky, and frustrated, Marsha asked me what was going on. After reviewing three days of daily food intake, Marsha was consuming almost twice as many calories from carbohydrates as she normally would eat to soothe her hunger pangs (and cravings) resulting from the drastic drop in her fat consumption.

If you astutely read the previous chapter, you would have the answer to this chapter's question: "Does fat make you fat?" Remember, any excess calorie that is not used or stored as energy is converted into excess body weight, including fat or adipose tissue. Just as dietary protein does not convert to the equivalent amount of muscle tissue, eating fat does not turn into fat tissue. However, eating excessive calories from foods containing fat, protein, or carbohydrates will.

Are fats from food bad for us? They are not. Like protein and carbohydrates, fats are an essential macronutrient. Dietary fats provide essential fatty acids (EFAs), carry fat-soluble vitamins, make hormones, and provide calories for energy. Fat is a concentrated energy source, providing nine calories per gram compared to four calories per gram in carbohydrate and protein. No wonder high-fat foods are so high in calories, providing over twice the calories as carbohydrates and protein by weight.

Certain fats and oils contain types of fatty acids that are good for our health. These are unsaturated fats, specifically monounsaturated and polyunsaturated fats. Unsaturated fats should replace saturated fats in our diet. Saturated fats have been shown to raise blood cholesterol levels. High blood cholesterol levels increase cardiovascular disease. However, most recent evidence pertaining to saturated fats is controversial. The evidence suggesting that dietary intake of saturated fats increase risk of cardiovascular disease is not uniformly supported.[91]

This reinforces the position that diet as a whole, not just one or two of its components, affects health. This could explain the long-standing French paradox. The French consume high amounts of saturated fat in cheese, pastries, butter, and sauces. However, the balance of their unsaturated fat intake along with other features of their diet and lifestyle affect their health. Butter and pastries are not the sole culprit.

Experts know with more certainty that high blood cholesterol levels are strongly linked to atherosclerosis or hardening of the arteries leading to heart disease, still the nation's number-one cause of morbidity and mortality. Arteries are the plumbing of our bodies' circulation, carrying blood and oxygen away from the heart to nourish our brain, organs, and other tissue in our bodies. When "bad" or low-density lipoprotein (LDL) cholesterol becomes oxidized, it can cause damage and inflammation to the lining of the arteries. When LDL cholesterol is too high, the likelihood of arterial damage increases.

Blood cholesterol levels should be routinely checked as part of your physical health exam. Below is the National Cholesterol Education Program's (NCEP) targets for blood fats, also called lipid profile. The NCEP recommends that all adults twenty years of age or older have a fasting lipid profile, which measures total cholesterol, LDL (bad) cholesterol, high-density lipoprotein (HDL, or good) cholesterol and triglycerides—once every five years or as directed by your physician based on lipid profile results.[92]

**Table 4.1: Components of Blood Lipid Profile and Their Target Values (Source: NCEP)**

| Component | Target (mg/dl) |
|---|---|
| Total blood cholesterol: | <200 |
| Low-density lipoprotein, or LDL ("bad blood cholesterol"): | <129 |
| High-density lipoprotein, or HDL ("good blood cholesterol"): | > or = 60 |
| Triglycerides: | <150 |

The blood lipid profile reveals much more about your risk for cardiovascular disease compared to a sole total cholesterol number. Physicians are able to review this panel of blood lipids to get a more accurate picture of your heart disease risk profile and blood lipid goals.

Just as a low total blood cholesterol level does not necessarily indicate a favorable heart disease risk profile, high total blood cholesterol does not mean you are at high risk of heart disease. A fit and healthy tennis friend of mine, Betsey, who recently turned sixty years old, realized the significance of her lipid profile numbers. Ironically, after her term life insurance policy penalized her for having a high total blood cholesterol, Betsey, the picture of health, curiously investigated. When her physician told Betsey her total blood cholesterol was 272 mg/dl, way above the 200 mg/dl target, she was dismayed.

He calmed her when he revealed her blood lipid profile. Betsey's LDL cholesterol was 125 mg/dl, and her HDL cholesterol was a mind-boggling, enviable 135 mg/dl. She proudly declared that her physician had never seen such a high "good" cholesterol level. Betsey's high total cholesterol number actually translated into a lipid profile indicating reduced cardiovascular risk.

Betsey is the poster child for healthy living. Betsey's lifestyle truly reflects the direct influence of diet and exercise on blood lipid levels. Betsey eats mostly fish, beans, whole grains, and nuts for protein. She always has a plethora of fresh vegetables and fruits in her refrigerator. She adds her daily flax or chia seeds to oatmeal, salads, and yogurt. She loves avocados, using them in place of trans fat–laden margarine, cheese, and salty salad dressings. She indulges in a glass of pinot noir two to three times a week. Betsey's BMI is within normal limits. She plays singles tennis at an elite division for her tennis league, competing with women far younger than she.

## THE SKINNY ON SATURATED FAT

For decades, we have been led to believe that saturated fat in foods like meat, butter, and cheese is bad for our heart health. The theory is that saturated fat raises blood cholesterol levels. High blood cholesterol is one of several risk factors for heart disease, because it can damage the arteries with sticky streaks, or plaque.

Saturated fat raises both the "bad" blood level, or LDL cholesterol, and the "good" blood level, or HDL cholesterol. Since saturated fat raises both kinds of cholesterol (good and bad), it has both a negative and a positive effect on blood lipid levels.

The chemical composition of saturated fats causes them to remain solid at room temperature. Examples of saturated fats include the fat found in beef, veal, lamb, and pork; the skin and fat on and around poultry; and the fat found in whole milk and whole and 2 percent milk fat products, such as cheese, ice cream, sour cream, and yogurt.

If saturated fat has a neutral effect on blood cholesterol level, then why the war on meat, cheese, and butter? Most recent research indicates that the connection between saturated fat and heart disease is not as well established as thought. Two major published study reviews, including one in *Annals of Internal Medicine* led by experts at Cambridge University, showed that there was no significant evidence that saturated fat increased risk of heart disease.[93]

Still controversial and inconclusive, these study reviews do not mean consumers should stock their refrigerators with butter, T-bone steaks, and whole milk. It does mean these once-shunned foods can fit (they always could have) in the context of a heart healthy diet—a reminder, once again, that a healthy diet should be inclusive, not exclusive. These studies open the door to more inquiry reexamining the saturated fat and heart disease riddle.

Aside from animal fats, three plant sources provide saturated fats in our diet: palm oil, cocoa butter, and coconut oil. These fats are found in processed, packaged baked goods and candy bars. These oils impart a desirable texture to packaged foods, extend their shelf life, and are inexpensive. First thought to raise blood cholesterol because of their chemical structure, cocoa butter and palm oil have not been demonstrated to do so. Still, be wary of these fats if they are listed as the first three ingredients on the food label. They can be replaced by fats that we know are better for health.

## COCONUT OIL: VILLAIN OR DARLING?

Coconut oil has received recent attention—but not as the artery-clogging villain in movie theater popcorn. Coconut oil is extracted from the kernel or meat of mature coconuts. Coconut oil contains the saturated fat lauric acid. Lauric acid may increase HDL (good cholesterol) and LDL (bad cholesterol) but not negatively affect the ratio of the two. Lauric acid is a medium-chain triglyceride or MCT. MCTs bypass the liver and are quickly used by the body for energy.

Why the recent attention on coconut oil? Thomas Brenna, professor of nutrition at Cornell University, believes the unfavorable reputation of coconut oil has evolved because studies demonstrating its lipid-raising effect used partially hydrogenated coconut oil, not untreated, virgin coconut oil. The trans fats produced through the partial hydrogenation of coconut oil may be the cause of high cholesterol levels. The culprit could be in the processing of coconut oil and not the coconut oil itself.[94]

Manufacturers and proponents of coconut oil tout that it promotes weight loss, improves metabolism, and boosts immune function; all these claims have yet to be substantiated. However, when coconut oil is used to replace butter, cream, or hydrogenated oils containing saturated and trans fats used in cooking, baking, or as a spread, it becomes a vegetarian option to these traditional fat sources. Use virgin coconut oil rather than processed coconut oil, which can be high in trans fats and additives and low in antioxidants.

## HYDROGENATION AND TRANS FATS

A significant source of trans-fatty acids, or trans fats, in the American diet is from hydrogenated oils. There are two sources of trans fats in our diet: natural and artificial trans fats. Natural trans fats are found in the fatty parts of meat and dairy products. In contrast, food processing called hydrogenation produces artificial trans fats. Hydrogenation is the process of converting a liquid oil into a solid fat by the chemical addition of hydrogen to its carbon chain. *Trans* refers to the physical positioning of hydrogen around the structure of the fatty acid. The food industry uses hydrogenated oils high in trans fats to improve the texture, shelf life, and flavor stability of foods.

Processed foods containing hydrogenated oils are a significant contributor of trans fats in the American diet. Approximately half the trans fats consumed by Americans are from hydrogenated oils in processed foods like crackers, snack chips, and margarine.[95] Studies show that trans fats raise total blood cholesterol. Trans fats raise LDL (bad) cholesterol and lower HDL (good) cholesterol. They are unequivocally bad for our health.

There are many processed foods containing trans fats. They include commercially baked goods, such as cookies, pies, and doughnuts; fast foods, such as french fries and fried chicken; stick margarine and shortening; and nondairy coffee creamers. To identify them on the ingredient label, look for hydrogenated oil, partially hydrogenated vegetable oil, or partially hydrogenated oil. Compared to the recent ambivalence about saturated fat, trans fats are a clear-cut nemesis to our heart health.

The food industry is working on ways to eliminate or reduce trans fats in processed foods. Since 2005, the amount of trans fat added to our food supply has declined by over 50 percent.[96] In

2006, the Food and Drug Administration (FDA), which regulates America's food labeling, has required manufacturers to identify trans fat content in packaged food products on the nutrition facts of the food label. Labels now identify trans fat content per serving of food items under the total fat content. To be considered trans fat–free, the item must contain under 0.5 grams of trans fat per serving.

Most recently, in the fall of 2013, the FDA announced a ban on artificial trans fats. This ban would require the food industry to gradually phase out all trans fats in their products, determining that partially hydrogenated oils are no longer "generally recognized as safe" (GRAS). The FDA's GRAS list consists of hundreds of food additives, such as colors and preservatives. Understanding their deleterious impact on public health, artificial trans fats will no longer be on the GRAS list.

Not confined to food manufacturing, the restaurant industry has taken a stand against serving trans fats in their establishments. New York City, Boston, Philadelphia, and the entire state of California have banned trans fats from their restaurant menus. Even entire countries have banned trans fats from their restaurants, including Denmark and Switzerland.

Not all restaurants have been as aggressive in removing trans fats from their menu items. Many fast-food chains still provide menu fare high in trans fats. One order of large fries in certain fast-food chains contains up to 5 grams of trans fats, exceeding the daily limit for most people. Since there are no trans fat labeling regulations for fast-food and other restaurants, be very discriminating about your menu selections. Take steps to ask the restaurant staff if they use trans fats in their menu items.

Fast-food restaurants appeal to children, teens, and young adults—tennis players on the rise. Some children consume as many fast-food meals as those eaten at the dinner table at home. Because food eaten away from home, including fast food, is a significant source of daily calories, knowing the nutritional content of these foods is vital.

Most fast-food restaurants make their nutritional information public. If nutritional guides cannot be found at the fast-food establishment, they are often available on the restaurant's website. Although a number of prominent fast-food chains have eliminated artificial trans fats in their menus, the overall nutrition in many of these foods is still far less than desirable.

## GUIDELINES FOR DIETARY FAT: QUALITY VERSUS QUANTITY

A far cry from the "no fat" and "fat phobia" in decades past, current research suggests consuming fats in proper proportion to promote heart health. Simply avoiding certain foods or nutrients will not lead to better health if the diet as a whole is inadequate. This same premise applies to fat. A low-fat diet is not necessarily healthy if the rest of the diet does not contain a healthy balance of nutrients.

*Two Cases in Point: the Mediterranean Diet and "Clean Diet" Philosophy.* Why has the world focused its attention on the Mediterranean diet? Diets based on cultural patterns of eating rather than on specific foods lead to health. The Mediterranean diet is a perfect example of a cultural eating pattern promoting cardiovascular health. Many experts regard the Mediterranean diet as the near-perfect eating plan,[97] and studies prove it. One well-known study found that three years on a Mediterranean diet reduced the subjects' risk of heart attack by up to 70 percent.[98] To promote the positive health benefits of the Mediterranean diet, many images including the Mediterranean diet food pyramid depict its dietary recommendations.

The Mediterranean diet includes a variety of fats from healthy food sources such as nuts, olives, fish, and seeds. This diet is also rich in antioxidant-packed vegetables and fruits. Seafood and fish are prepared with olive or canola oil and served with whole grains or minimally processed grains. Meat and dairy are consumed in small portions. Water and red wine are the staple beverages of the Mediterranean diet. Portion size is under control at each meal, while physical exercise is liberal. Meals are events, enjoyed and savored at the table with family and friends. Exercise and activity are a daily part of the Mediterranean lifestyle. This cultural pattern markedly contrasts to the fast-paced, supersized Western diet and lifestyle.

Another dietary pattern involves clean eating. The philosophy of clean eating has been around for a while but has reemerged in popularity. Clean eating encourages eaters to

- choose whole, unprocessed foods, such as fruits, vegetables, and grains, avoiding highly processed, genetically modified, and refined foods;
- eat a varied diet;
- use locally grown and seasonal foods, thereby reducing the environmental impact or "carbon" footprint; and
- take the time to enjoy food at mealtimes.[99]

Like the Mediterranean diet, the clean movement is an eating pattern that focuses on many aspects of healthful eating. Notice these healthy patterns do not focus on limiting or excluding one or more foods or food groups, like so many fad diets do.

Lessons learned from the Mediterranean diet have caused experts to more closely examine dietary guidelines for Americans. The principles from this eating pattern are very much aligned with those suggested by leading nutrition and health professionals. The Mediterranean diet still restricts saturated fat, replacing it with healthy fats like monounsaturated fats and omega-3s. Although the Western eating pattern does not mirror the Mediterranean diet, the American Heart Association's Nutrition Committee supports similar dietary fat guidelines for healthy Americans over the age of two:

- Limit total fat intake to less than 25–35 percent of your total calories each day. (The 2010 dietary guidelines, the Academy of Nutrition and Dietetics, and the World Health Organization/Food and Agricultural Organization recommend less than 20–35 percent of your total calories come from fat.)
- Limit saturated fat intake to less than 7 percent of total daily calories each day.
- Limit trans fat intake to less than 1 percent of total daily calories each day.
- The remaining fat should come from sources of monounsaturated and polyunsaturated fats, such as nuts, seeds, fish, and vegetable oils.
- Limit cholesterol intake to fewer than 300 milligrams per day. If you have heart disease or your LDL cholesterol level is 100 mg/dl or greater, limit cholesterol intake to less than 200 milligrams per day.[100]

## IT'S A BALANCING ACT: OMEGA-6 AND OMEGA-3 FATS

Unsaturated fats should replace saturated fats—*in the proper balance*. The two types of unsaturated fats are polyunsaturated and monounsaturated fats. Monounsaturated fatty acids (MUFAs)—which are found in olive, canola (rapeseed), peanut, and avocado oil—have been shown to benefit blood cholesterol levels and heart health. When MUFAs replace saturated fats in our diet, they may decrease total blood cholesterol levels while maintaining HDL, or "good," blood cholesterol level.

Polyunsaturated fatty acids (PUFAs) have been shown to

lower total blood cholesterol. PUFAs lower both HDL ("good" cholesterol) and LDL ("bad" cholesterol) levels.

PUFAs include the families called omega-6 and omega-3 fatty acids. Linoleic acid, a type of omega-6 fatty acid, is found in vegetable sources like soybean, corn, cottonseed, and safflower oil. These oils are used to make salad dressings, margarine, and mayonnaise, common food sources of linoleic acid in our diet. Fried food in restaurants or in the home is more than likely steeped in vegetable oils high in PUFAs. Look on a bag of potato chips, and chances are cottonseed, peanut, or sunflower oil is the second ingredient behind potatoes. Less common sources of PUFAs, such as arachidonic acid, come from meat and egg yolks.

There are two main sources of omega-3 fatty acids: animal and plant sources. Animal sources of omega-3 fatty acids most commonly include cold-water fatty fish, such as salmon and mackerel. These fatty fish contain the omega-3 fatty acids called EPA and DHA—helpful abbreviations for eicosapenteanoic acid and docosahexaenoic acid. EPA and DHA come from animal sources and promote heart health.

Grass-fed beef is also a good source of omega-3 fatty acids, much higher in EPA and DHA than grain-fed beef. Food industrialization has changed even what our livestock consumes. Because corn is a highly subsidized and affordable crop, farmers readily use corn for animal feed rather than grass. When cows eat corn rather than grass, the composition of beef changes. The result is beef with a much lower EPA and DHA content. The price tag will reflect this difference. In most supermarkets, you now must pay a premium price for grass-fed beef versus grain- or corn-fed beef.

Another type of omega-3 fatty acid, called alpha-linolenic acid (ALA), is found in plant sources, such as flaxseeds, chia seeds, almonds, pistachios, and walnuts. ALA is also good for heart health. Flaxseeds and chia seeds have become appealing additions to many foods for this beneficial reason.

# THE POWER OF FLAX AND CHIA SEEDS

Flaxseeds and chia seeds are tiny but pack a powerful nutrient punch. Comparing the nutrition between these superstar seeds is analogous to Roger Federer and Novak Djokovic battling it out in a Grand Slam final. These superfood seeds owe their nutritional merit to lignan, fiber, protein, calcium, and omega-3 fatty acids.

Lignan is a type of phytoestrogen, a plant chemical with weak estrogen effects. Phytoestrogens (also found in whole soy foods like tofu, soy milk, and soy nuts) may aid in the prevention of hormone-related cancer, such as breast or prostate cancer. Lignan also acts as a potent antioxidant. Flaxseeds are higher in lignan content than chia seeds.

Two tablespoons of flaxseeds provide 3.2 grams or 3,200 milligrams of the omega-3 fatty acid ALA, exceeding the recommended amount for the entire day. The same amount of chia seeds offers slightly less ALA. If you cannot get two tablespoons of flax or chia seeds in your daily diet, you can also get ALA from almonds and walnuts.

The valuable nutrients in flaxseeds are significantly more bioavailable when flaxseeds are crushed. This is because whole flaxseeds will pass through you, undigested. Choose ground flaxseeds to reap their nutritional benefit. Store them in the refrigerator to prevent oxidation of their valuable fatty acids. Refrigeration keeps ground flaxseeds from becoming rancid.

Chia seeds are the same seeds that create the furry green iconic Chia Pets. Who would have "thunk"? Unlike flaxseeds that need to be crushed, the nutrition in whole chia seeds is readily bioavailable. Therefore, chia seeds can be eaten either whole or crushed.

Like flaxseeds, chia seeds also have superfood star quality. Chia seeds have the unique quality of being a plant source containing complete protein. This means chia seeds contain all essential amino acids. Chia seeds also have more calcium than flaxseeds. Like flaxseeds, chia seeds are rich in ALA. Chia seeds are higher in antioxidant content than flaxseeds, which causes them to stay fresh and store longer than flaxseeds. Chia seeds have a more neutral flavor compared to flaxseeds and can be sprinkled on salads, cereals, and baked products. When left in water, chia seeds form a gel that can be used in place of eggs, oil, or butter in cooking.

Fuel your tennis nutrition by using these tips to incorporate chia seeds in your diet:

- ✓ use as a thickening agent for soups, gravies, sauces, jams, and puddings or a binding agent for meatballs
- ✓ mix with water as a substitute for eggs in baked recipes
- ✓ add to oatmeal, salads, granola, and fruit crisps
- ✓ use as a breading for fish, chicken, and tofu

So, which seed wins the nutritional throw down? Chia seeds edge flaxseeds. But because each contributes such emphatically good nutrition, both can easily be incorporated into a healthy diet.

**Table 4.2: Food Sources of Omega Fats**

| Omega Family | Types of Fat | Food Sources |
| --- | --- | --- |
| Omega-6 | Linoleic acid | Peanut, soybean, sunflower, corn, safflower, grapeseed, cottonseed oils. Mayonnaise, salad dressing, margarine |
| | Arachidonic Acid | Meat, egg yolks |
| Omega-3 | Alpha-linolenic acid, or ALA | Flaxseeds, chia seeds, walnuts, hemp, canola oil, pumpkin seeds |
| | EPA and DHA | Cold-water fatty fish (e.g., salmon, mackerel), algae, grass-fed meat |

When it comes to dietary fat, quality is as important as quantity. The evolving Western diet is now prolific with the omega-6 fatty acid, linoleic acid, and low in omega-3 fatty acids. This dietary fat profile appears to be proinflammatory and disease promoting. Chronic inflammation is best understood in relation to cardiovascular disease.

When blood vessels are besieged by oxidized LDL, or "bad," cholesterol, white blood cells from our immune system gobble up the LDL cholesterol, all the while causing damage to arteries. Over time—weeks, months, and years—the chronic inflammatory process that tries to heal damages the lining of the arteries of the heart at the same time. These destructive reactions that damage cells lead to cardiovascular disease or atherosclerosis.

Chronic inflammation, which experts concur causes disease onset and progression, should not be confused with acute inflammation. In acute inflammation, the immune system works rapidly to heal an injury. A cut on your finger, a burn, an ankle sprain, or a muscle strain elicit a rapid cascade of inflammatory events. Analogous to an army of rescue soldiers, acute inflammation causes a release of healing white blood cells. Acute inflammation also causes an increase in blood flow and permeability to ensure oxygen and nutrients are delivered to the injury as quickly as possible. Ever sprained your ankle in a tennis fall? That bruised, puffy, and reddened tenderness in your ankle is the thankful result of acute inflammation. Acute inflammation is desirable; chronic inflammation is not.

Chronic or systemic inflammation is the root cause of several diseases, such as rheumatoid arthritis, lupus, and the inflammatory bowel diseases, Crohn's disease, and ulcerative colitis. Could it also be the cause of many common diseases in the Western world, such as cancer, heart disease, Alzheimer's disease, stroke, and diabetes? Research is fervently working on whether chronic inflammation plays a role in these common diseases that plague Americans.

What does dietary fat have to do with inflammation? With the industrialization in the food industry, liquid vegetable oils, mayonnaise, margarines, and packaged, processed foods have become commonplace in our kitchen cupboards and refrigerators. The increased consumption of these types of fat has resulted in an all-time high amount of omega-6s in our diet. These omega-6s have replaced the blood cholesterol–raising saturated fat in solid fats—the type of fat Americans were told to limit. Manufacturers have ensured their labels state "Made with Vegetable Oil." But a product is not always healthful just because the term *vegetable* is on it—unhealthy, trans fat–laden partially hydrogenated vegetable oil is a reminder of this. In addition, the chemical structure of omega-6s themselves are very subject to reacting with oxygen, producing harmful free radicals that can lead to oxidative cellular damage.

Omega-6s need to be in proper balance with omega-3 fatty acids to produce a more desirable heart-health ratio. Currently, Americans eat a fat profile ratio at an all-time high of 20–30:1 omega-6s:omega-3s. The desirable ratio is 4:1. The current American diet has over four times the amount of omega-6s to omega-3s, creating a proinflammatory dietary fat profile.[101] To get this ratio back in line, incorporate the following guidelines:

1. Replace saturated fats with monounsaturated fats (MUFAs) and polyunsaturated fats (PUFAs). Substitute soybean, corn, and safflower oils and mayonnaise, margarine, and salad dressings made with these oils or with olive, canola, avocado, walnut, sesame, or peanut oils.

2. Increase omega-3 fatty acids by getting daily doses of plant and marine sources. Get EPA and DHA from two to three servings of cold-water fatty fish per week.

Examples of cold-water fish include the following:

| | |
|---|---|
| Alaskan wild salmon | Sablefish/black cod |
| Arctic char | Anchovies |
| Mackerel | Rainbow trout |
| Sardines | Albacore tuna |

Be reminded fatty cold-water fish can be high in mercury, PCB, and other toxins. Also, for the environmentally friendly fish eater, look for fish caught through sustainable seafood practices.

Get ALA from plant sources. Sources of ALA include the following:

| | |
|---|---|
| Walnuts and walnut oil | Canola oil |
| Chia seeds | Soybeans and soybean oil |
| Flaxseeds | Perilla seed oil |
| Hemp seed oil | Pumpkin seeds and pumpkin seed oil |

Add these ALA-rich foods to yogurt and salads. Grind flaxseeds to improve their omega-3 fatty acid availability. Otherwise, we pass them undigested without reaping their health benefits.

Making anti-inflammatory dietary changes can actually be tracked in your blood. Your physician can monitor and evaluate the levels of the inflammatory marker in your blood called C-reactive protein. This is a measure of how changes in diet and lifestyle, including dietary fat profile, can affect inflammatory response.

Aside from a desirable dietary fat profile, there are other features of an anti-inflammatory diet. Experts suggest the following:

- Increase vegetables and fruits to at least eight to ten servings per day—they contain polyphenols, which show potent anti-inflammatory effect. Other foods with polyphenols include dark chocolate, coffee, and tea.
- Cook with olive oil as much as possible.
- Eat plenty of foods with vitamins E and C, which may boost the immune system. Citrus fruits, kiwi, strawberries, bell peppers, and tomatoes are a few foods rich in vitamin C. Be sure to get vitamin E from its gamma-tocopherol form, found in nuts, seeds, and vegetable oils, and its alpha-tocopherol form in vitamin E supplements.
- Eat whole grains. Replace refined, processed grains with whole grains.
- Eat more foods containing omega-3 fatty acids, such as salmon, chia seeds, flaxseeds, walnuts, and canola oil.
- Include foods containing prebiotics and probiotics. Prebiotics are in onions, bananas, garlic, asparagus, chicory, and jerusalem artichokes. Probiotics are in cultured dairy foods like yogurt and kefir. Both appear to show anti-inflammatory effects in the digestive tract.
- Decrease intake of trans fats that are in many processed and fast foods.
- Cut down on sugary foods like sodas, candy, cakes, and cookies.[102]

Notice a common theme? Fruits, vegetables, whole grains, and a proper balance of dietary fats are key to decreasing disease and promoting health. Although the final word is out on whether an anti-inflammatory diet can conclusively reduce risk of chronic disease, many of the characteristics of an anti-inflammatory diet show favorable evidence. Plus, you cannot go wrong with its guidelines for overall good nutrition.

Using the NCEP recommendations, you can calculate suggested fat intake and then incorporate suggested types of fat in the proper amounts and ratios to match the quantity with the quality of dietary fat intake. Using a total of 1,800 calories per day, fat intake should be the following:

**Total Fat:**
1.  35 percent of total calories from fat
    1,800 calories per day × 35 percent of calories from fat = 630 calories from fat.

    630 calories from fat per day ÷ 9 calories per 1 gram of fat = 70 grams of fat per day. (Note that 1,800 calories a day may be a typical calorie requirement for a female club player. Competitive, trained players may need two or even three times this number of calories each day.)

2.  25 percent of total calories from fat
    1,800 calories per day × 25 percent of calories from fat = 450 calories from fat.

    450 calories from fat per day ÷ 9 calories per 1 gram of fat = 50 grams of fat per day.

**Saturated Fat:**
1800 calories per day × 7 percent of calories from saturated fat = 126 calories from saturated fat, or 14 grams of saturated fat, per day. Be sure to include saturated fat as part of the total fat figure, not in addition to it.

**Trans Fat:**
1,800 calories per day × 1 percent of calories from trans fats = 18 calories, or 2 grams, of trans fats per day. This is a very small allowance due to the trans fats' damaging cardiovascular impact. Like saturated fat, this amount is included in the total daily fat intake.

> **Dietary fat intake profile based on 1,800 calories/day**
> Total fat: 50–70 g per day
> Saturated fat: <14 g per day
> Trans fat: <2 g per day
> 4:1 omega-6:omega-3 ratio: 7.2 g (7,200 mg): 1.8 g (1,800 mgs)

Saturated fat and trans fats should be replaced by unsaturated fats with omega-6s and omega-3s in the proper ratio of 4:1.[103]

You may think that the above calculations result in a large allotment of total fat grams for the day, but look how much fat is in a typical American breakfast—a breakfast that many children, teen, or adult tennis players consume.

**Table 4.3: Fat Content of an Unhealthy Breakfast**

| Item | Total Fat (g) | Saturated Fat (g) | Trans Fat (g) |
|---|---|---|---|
| 2 scrambled eggs, fried in | 10 | 3.2 | 0 |
| 1 tablespoon stick margarine | 10 | 7 | 3 |
| 1 large cake doughnut | 22 | 10 | 5 |
| 2 slices bacon | 7 | 2 | 0 |
| 1 cup coffee w/ 2 tablespoons half-and-half | 4 | 2 | 0 |
| **Total Fat:** | **53** | **24 .2** | **8** |

Eating 53 grams of fat in one meal is more than the total suggested lower limit of fat for an *entire day* on an 1,800-calorie-per-day menu. Eating 24.2 grams of saturated fat and 8 grams of trans fat in this unhealthy breakfast meal also exceeds the suggested limit in an entire day.

The high saturated and trans fat content is not the only dietary disaster in this menu. This meal is low in desirable omega-3 fats, fiber, vitamins, and phytonutrients from fruits and whole grains. What can be done to modify this breakfast train wreck? The below menu replaces saturated fat with healthy unsaturated fats and improves the ratio of omega-6 to omega-3 fatty acids by adding a good dose of ALA. Review the nutritious and delicious breakfast makeover below.

**Table 4.4: Fat Content of a Healthy Breakfast**

| Item | Total Fat (g) | Saturated Fat (g) | Trans Fat (g) | Omega- 3 Fats (mg) | MUFAs (g) |
|---|---|---|---|---|---|
| 1 hard-boiled egg, omega 3-enriched | 5.6 | 1.6 | 0 | 450 | 2 |
| 1 cup cooked oatmeal w/ 1 tablespoon dried cherries and 1 tablespoon brown sugar | 3 | .5 | 0 | 90 | 1 |
| 1 tablespoon ground flaxseeds | 3 | 0 | 0 | 1,600 | .5 |
| 6 ounces calcium-fortified orange juice | 0 | 0 | 0 | 0 | 0 |
| 1 cup coffee | 0 | 0 | 0 | 0 | 0 |
| 2 tablespoons fat-free evaporated milk | 0 | 0 | 0 | 0 | 0 |
| **Total Fat** | **11.6** | **2.1** | **0** | **2,140** | **3.5** |

The difference in total fat content, fat profile, calories, and nutrition between these two breakfasts is remarkable. The typical American breakfast in the first menu is laden with fat and calories and devoid of omega-3 fatty acids, MUFAs, fiber, and antioxidants. This menu needs a nutritional overhaul. In its nutrition makeover, menu two provides antioxidant-rich dried cherries, whole-grain oatmeal, and high-quality egg protein, creating a much healthier breakfast plate. A generous dose of flaxseeds provides omega-3 fatty acids (ALA) and lignan. In menu two, calcium-fortified orange juice provides calcium as well as folate and vitamin C. Wiser food choices result in big gains in nutrition—and tennis performance.

## DIETARY CHOLESTEROL: THE EGG UPDATE

Eggs were used in the above menu example for a reason. The AHA suggests keeping dietary cholesterol intake to fewer than 300 milligrams per day. Cholesterol is found in foods of animal origin, such as eggs, whole-milk dairy products and meat, poultry, and shellfish. One large egg contains approximately 250 milligrams of dietary cholesterol—almost the full day's limit for cholesterol. No wonder eggs have received the stamp of disapproval for their high cholesterol content.

However, the unfavorable reputation of eggs has not been supported by fact. Studies have yet to show that egg consumption is associated with higher blood cholesterol levels in human populations.[104] Dietary cholesterol has relatively little effect on blood cholesterol compared to saturated and trans fats.

Eggs are very nutritious, containing high-quality, high-biological-value (HBV) protein, iron, zinc, vitamins B12, B6, A, D, and E, biotin, choline, and the carotenoid antioxidants lutein and zeaxanthin. Lutein and zeaxanthin may keep eyes healthy by reducing age-related macular degeneration. Pastured eggs and omega-3 eggs are even more nutritious than conventional eggs.

Omega-3 eggs owe their favorable fat profile to their chickens whose feed is supplemented with high omega-3 sources like flaxseeds. Some feel eggs are so nutritious they are worthy of superfood status.

The AHA no longer has the "three eggs per week" limit it used to religiously prescribe. Adhering to the belief that all foods can fit in a healthy eating pattern, the AHA does not endorse consuming or avoiding eggs. Consume eggs in line with the NCEP's dietary guidelines for total daily fat and cholesterol intake to reap the nutritional benefit of one of nature's superfoods. The complete makeover of menu one produces the super nutrition in menu two.

| Unhealthy Menu | Healthy Menu Makeover |
|---|---|
| Menu One | Menu Two |
| BREAKFAST | BREAKFAST |
| 2 scrambled eggs (fried in 1 tablespoon margarine)<br>1 large cake doughnut<br>2 slices bacon<br>1 cup coffee with half-and-half | 1 hard-boiled egg<br>1 cup oatmeal w/<br>1 tablespoon dried cherries and<br>1 tablespoon ground flaxseeds<br>1 tablespoon brown sugar<br>6 ounces calcium-fortified orange juice<br>1 cup coffee w/ 2 tablespoons fat-free evaporated milk |
| SNACK | SNACK |
| 1-1 ounce bag potato chips | 6 ounces vanilla greek yogurt<br>1 small banana |
| LUNCH | LUNCH |
| 4 ounce cheeseburger, ground chuck w/ 1 slice American processed cheese<br>ketchup, mustard, mayonnaise<br>6 onion rings<br>1-20 ounce bottle of soda | 3 ounce black-bean burger<br>1 whole-grain bun<br>lettuce, tomato, onion, ketchup<br>1 ounce sweet-potato chips<br>1 medium apple<br>water |

| Unhealthy Menu | Healthy Menu Makeover |
|---|---|
| Menu One | Menu Two |
| DINNER | DINNER |
| 1 cup macaroni and cheese<br>1/2 cup canned green beans<br>1 two-inch brownie<br>1-16 ounce bottle of sports drink | 3 ounces baked wild salmon<br>w/ 1 cup spring mix salad,<br>tomatoes, carrots, red pepper,<br>edamame, and garbanzo beans<br>2 tablespoons vinegar and olive<br>oil dressing<br>1 cup brown rice<br>1 whole-fruit strawberry<br>frozen bar<br>water |
| SNACK | SNACK |
| 1 ounce pretzels | 1 cup of whole-grain cereal with 1 cup soy, almond, skim, or 1 percent milk, 1/2 cup blueberries |

Like its breakfast menu, menu one is high in saturated and trans fats, low in calcium and vitamin D, low in both MUFAs and omega-3 fatty acids, high in simple sugar, and low in fiber and phytonutrients due to its dearth of whole grains and fresh fruits and vegetables. Menu one is representative of a day's worth of tragic eating for many, including athletes on the tennis court.

In contrast, menu two provides nutrients, vitamins, minerals, fiber, antioxidants, and fats in the proper portion sizes and ratios from healthy food sources. Take a close look at menu two to obtain ideas on how to provide nutritional potency to your food selection. You will feel the difference high-energy eating makes on the tennis court.

# THE FOOD LABEL

If you need an immediate guide to good eating, the food label can be a quick and effective resource. Since its inception over twenty years ago, the FDA has made the nutrition facts of the food label more user-friendly. The nutrition facts portion of the food label is a quick, handy reference, distinguishing fat content in packaged foods. Under total fat content, the nutrition facts will specify the amount of saturated fat, trans fat, and unsaturated fat per serving of the food item. The food label also lists cholesterol, sodium, total carbohydrates, and protein.

The percentage daily value based on two thousand calories per day is listed to the right of each nutrient. Daily values (DV) are nutritional targets for food labeling purpose. They help put a particular food in context of a total daily diet. The DV is not the same as the RDA, but it does incorporate the RDA for its figures based off two thousand calories per day. Table 4.5 lists the DV for food labeling.

**Table 4.5: Daily Values for Nutrients on the Food Label (Source: FDA)**

| Food Component | DV |
| --- | --- |
| Total Fat | 65 grams (g) |
| Saturated Fat | 20 g |
| Cholesterol | 300 milligrams (mg) |
| Sodium | 2,400 mg |
| Potassium | 3,500 mg |
| Total Carbohydrate | 300 g |
| Dietary Fiber | 25 g |
| Protein | 50 g |
| Vitamin A | 5,000 international units (IU) |

| Food Component | DV |
|---|---|
| Vitamin C | 60 mg |
| Calcium | 1,000 mg |
| Iron | 18 mg |
| Vitamin D | 400 IU |
| Vitamin E | 30 IU |
| Vitamin K | 80 micrograms (µg) |
| Thiamin | 1.5 mg |
| Riboflavin | 1.7 mg |
| Niacin | 20 mg |
| Vitamin B6 | 2 mg |
| Folate | 400 µg |
| Vitamin B12 | 6 µg |
| Biotin | 300 µg |
| Pantothenic acid | 10 mg |
| Phosphorus | 1,000 mg |
| Iodine | 150 µg |
| Magnesium | 400 mg |
| Zinc | 15 mg |
| Selenium | 70 µg |
| Copper | 2 mg |
| Manganese | 2 mg |
| Chromium | 120 µg |
| Molybdenum | 75 µg |
| Chloride | 3,400 mg |

The label provides the percentage of the daily value that a serving size of the food item provides. Interpreting percentage of daily values takes a little help from some grade-school math. Here are some examples:

- A portion of cheese provides 20 percent of the daily value for calcium.
- The daily value for calcium is 1,000 milligrams.
- The amount in the serving size would have 200 milligrams of calcium (20 percent of 1000 milligrams).

Sample information from the food label for a bag of potato chips is shown below.

Serving Size: 1 oz. (28 g / About 15 potato chips)

| | |
|---|---|
| Calories 160 | Calories from Fat 90 |
| Total Fat | 10 g |
|     Saturated Fat | 1 g |
|     Trans Fat | 0 g |
|     Polyunsaturated Fat | 2.5 g |
|     Monounsaturated Fat | 5 g |
| Sodium | 160 mg |

Ingredients: Potatoes, Vegetable Oil (Sunflower, Corn, and/or Canola Oil), Salt. No Preservatives.

Listed on the top of the nutrition facts, the serving size identifies the portion from which the nutrients and percentage daily values are based. When reviewing the food label, always identify the serving size first. A twenty-ounce bottle of regular soda may appear to be one serving, while its label reveals that it is actually one and a half servings. By drinking the whole soda, you consume even more sugar than what's listed on the food label. Double up nutrition in healthy foods, not through sugar-laden soda.

In the above example, the serving size is one ounce, or fifteen potato chips. The nutrition facts are based on this serving size— no more, no less. Not surprisingly, over two-thirds of the calories in a serving of potato chips are from fat. Since a high fat content is to be expected of all fried foods, focus on the types of fat the food item provides. In this example, the total fat breaks down to the following profile:

1 g of fat is from saturated fat
2.5 g of fat are from PUFAs
5 g of fat are from MUFAs
0 g of fat are from trans fats

The numbers may not always add up to the total fat content, because they are rounded up or down.

Is this healthy chip an oxymoron? Although the majority of calories are from fat, there are no trans fats and minimal saturated fat, with more MUFAs than PUFAs. Even the sodium content in this serving of chips is reasonable. Reading the ingredient label, there are no additives and preservatives. The vegetable oil source is listed as a combination of corn, safflower, and canola oil. This product deserves a thumbs-up on nutritional profile—for potato chips.

The FDA has recently proposed to update the nutrition facts label to help consumers make more informed decisions about the food they eat. Several pending changes include the following:[105]

- Establish more realistic serving sizes to reflect how much people typically eat at one time. Over the decades, this portion size has ballooned. For example, the current food label typically has a half cup of ice cream as a serving size, when most people typically eat at least twice that amount. The proposed new serving size would be one cup of ice cream. Similarly, package sizes have also expanded so that a twenty-ounce beverage, which most people will drink in a single setting, will equal one serving.

  A logical criticism of this labeling change is that just because these portion sizes are more realistic does not mean that they should be the norm. A twenty-ounce soda is still twenty ounces too many of empty calories. Remember, the food label is based on one serving size. If a large serving size is consumed, so are its excess calories, fat and sodium. When the new labeling changes take place, tread carefully, making sure you understand that these portions may be large. The nutrition facts on the label will reflect this.

- Calories and serving size will be more prominent to better grasp the attention of eaters who are watching their weight—one effort to address the overweight and obesity public health concern.

- Provide updated information on the latest nutritional science findings. Daily values for nutrients like sodium, fiber, and vitamin D will be updated. The new label will require more information on "Added Sugars," knowing that refined sugar added to foods equates to additional empty calories. It will keep total fat, saturated fat, and trans fat but remove "Calories from Fat." As discussed, research shows the type of fat is more important to our health than the amount.

Let's refer back to Marsha at the beginning of the chapter. She learned that both the type and total amount of fat in her diet influenced her health. A proper balance of the type of fat in her diet was key to healthy eating—not just the amount, a belief that was so prevalent in years past. The days of counting fat grams are over. Fat is one of three macronutrients essential in our diet. A healthy profile of fats provides a functional role in reducing inflammation and oxidative damage—the two primary causes of disease. Once Marsha understood that a healthy diet was inclusive of all foods, including fats, she began to lose the weight while making gains in her tennis game.

# 5

## CARBOHYDRATES: FRIEND, NOT FOE

**In my mind, I'm always the best. If I walk out on the court and think the next person is better, I've already lost.**
—Venus Williams

Andrew is a former professional tennis player and coach. His life and livelihood revolve around tennis. Andrew, a tall, muscular, and very fit thirtysomething, wanted to take his fitness to the next level by eliminating carbohydrates and consuming mostly protein in his diet. His daily lunches tirelessly consisted of two grilled chicken breasts and salad neatly packed in his plastic containers and securely tucked in his tennis bag. On occasion, Andrew would proudly show me his lunches—his discipline was inspiring. Andrew lost weight, got fit, and got back the six-pack abs he sported when he was on the tour. Problem: Andrew could not bear to eat chicken any longer and started to loathe his diet regimen. Incidentally, Andrew's weight loss was due to his intense training regimen coupled with the drastic reduction in total calories through his high-protein, low-carb diet—not as a direct result of low-carb diet.

# THE CARBOHYDRATE CONTROVERSY

Although the resurgent popularity of the high-protein, low-carbohydrate diet—in and out of our lives for decades—has diminished, its legacy lives on for many. That "carbohydrates are bad for you" is an erroneous oversimplification at its best. Other inaccurate statements I have commonly heard about carbohydrates include "Carbohydrates will make you fat ... make you have diabetes ... make you feel sluggish" and so on.

Carbohydrates are not only good for you, they are an essential macronutrient in our diet, just like protein and fat—and especially critical in providing the fuel necessary for peak tennis performance. Foods with carbohydrates also provide fiber, phytonutrients, vitamins, and minerals, including iron. We cannot live without carbohydrates. The body converts carbohydrates into glucose, providing our muscles and brain the fuel for daily activity and exercise. Carbohydrates also prevent muscle fatigue.

Nutrients like carbohydrates not only serve their essential role to nourish, they also enhance tennis sports performance. Think of carbohydrates as functional in your tennis game—a nutrient with a mission. Nutrition is a dynamically emerging field as sports scientists discover that foods and fluids serve an important function in improving athletic performance. Nutrition has been catapulted into the limelight for its starring role as "functional food," with carbohydrates being center stage for the athlete.

There are two types of carbohydrates—sugars and starches. Sugars are also referred to as simple carbohydrates. Starches are also referred to as complex carbohydrates. Sugars are more simple in chemical structure than starch, hence their name.

Simple sugars include the monosaccharides: glucose, galactose, and fructose. Monosaccharides contain one sugar unit. Disaccharides contain two sugar units and include sucrose (table sugar), maltose, and lactose (milk sugar). Polysaccharides are chains of monosaccharides, which contain more than ten sugar units. Examples of polysaccharides include starch and glycogen.

Foods high in simple sugars include candy, table sugar, honey, sugary beverages, and desserts. Many foods high in simple sugars are also high in saturated and trans fats, such as pies, cakes, ice cream, doughnuts, and pastries. These high-sugar foods contribute empty and excess calories, which can lead to weight gain, spikes in blood sugar, hyperinsulinemia (excessive production of insulin), and dental caries (tooth decay).

Empty calories come from foods that are nutrient poor. Eating empty calories is analogous to quantity without quality— foods high in calories and low in nutrition. As an example, one regular twelve-ounce can of soda contains 140 empty calories and 39 grams of simple sugar. This is the equivalent of nearly ten teaspoons of table sugar, although most soda no longer even contains table sugar or sucrose—it is high fructose corn syrup. A twenty-ounce bottle of soda contains 240 calories and 65 grams of simple sugar, equal to a whopping sixteen teaspoons of table sugar. Regular soda offers significant calories with no nutrition. As much as possible, avoid choosing foods with empty calories, many of which contain simple sugars, and replace them with healthier foods and beverages low in simple sugars.

While many sugary sodas, teas, and fruit drinks contain high fructose corn syrup, one popular sports drink still contains carbohydrate in the form of maltodextrin. Research has shown maltodextrin to be most effective sugar in quickly delivering the fuel necessary for optimal sports performance. Sports drinks are ergogenic beverages. They are engineered to provide the right type of simple sugar in the right amount to deliver fuel for the working muscles.

However, sports drinks should be used for the purpose they were designed—providing fast-acting carbohydrates during sustained exercise. If sports drinks have taken the place of healthier beverages like water or milk at the dinner table, they provide empty sugar calories, as well as unneeded sodium and artificial colors. (Chapter 7 further discusses sports drinks and their role in tennis hydration.)

If carbohydrates are essential in our diet, and especially important for tennis players, then what's fueling the carbohydrate controversy? Over the past thirty years, America's diet has dramatically changed. The percentage of calories from carbohydrates from simple sugars has increased while the percentage of calories from fat has declined.[106] Back when butter and red meat were taboo, one would think the experts touting the benefits of a low-fat diet would be pleased by this statistic. They would be, if the calories from fatty foods were either not replaced at all or replaced by healthier foods like vegetables, fruits, nuts, seeds, and whole grains. Instead, they have been replaced by sugary beverages and refined carbohydrates in sweets, crackers, and snack chips.

These carbohydrates, like all carbohydrates, are digested and turn into glucose or sugar in our blood. The presence of blood sugar stimulates our bodies to produce insulin. In contrast, when blood sugar is low, the body releases the hormone glucagon to raise blood sugar.

Insulin and glucagon maintain proper blood sugar levels necessary for the function of our brain, liver, and kidney. Insulin is the hormone produced by the islet cells in our pancreas. The pancreas is the organ located behind our stomach, surrounded by the small intestine, liver, and spleen. Insulin latches on to each molecule of blood sugar to quickly pull it into muscles and organs for use, as well as into fat tissue for storage.

When there is a constant surge of insulin to manage blood sugar from the excessive amounts of sugary carbohydrates we eat, the body is in a state of hyperinsulinemia. Hyperinsulinemia is the body's overcompensation of insulin production. This results in fat cells going into a fervent caloric storage overdrive.

When hyperinsulinemia quickly delivers these sugar calories into tissue, we may feel the urge to eat more, which results in more insulin being released. The vicious cycle ensues, eventually leading to a condition called insulin resistance, which causes weight gain, prediabetes, type 2 diabetes, and high blood triglyceride levels.

Prediabetes, familiarly coined as *borderline diabetes*, occurs when blood sugar is elevated but not high enough to be classified as diabetes. Prediabetes frequently leads to full-blown diabetes. Many active tennis players may believe that prediabetes and diabetes only happen to someone else, such as the elderly, obese, or sedentary individuals. The fact is that eighty-six million Americans over the age of twenty have prediabetes, almost one-fifth of the population. Less than 10 percent even realize they have prediabetes.[107]

Since your routine physical exam includes blood glucose as part of the laboratory's complete blood count (CBC), your blood glucose reading is accessible. Ask your physician for more information on your blood glucose reading. In addition, offer your MD your risk factors for prediabetes or diabetes, especially if you are elderly, overweight, and/or have a family history. Women who have had gestational diabetes, which is diabetes during pregnancy, are also at risk of developing diabetes later in life.

Unlike the empty calories found in sugary foods that should be kept to a minimum, many starchy foods are nutrient dense. Tennis players need these healthier carbohydrates for energy. Starchy foods like whole grains, beans, legumes, and certain vegetables contain high amounts of fiber, vitamins, and phytonutrients. Most sugary foods do not. Diets high in fiber have been shown to reduce blood cholesterol levels and aid digestion. Experts associate high-fiber diets (although have not proven) with lower rates of certain types of cancer.

What appears to fuel the carbohydrate controversy is the notion that all carbohydrates are "bad," when the root of the problem is the excessive amounts of simple sugars children, teens, and adults consume. Be sure to choose healthier carbs over simple carbohydrates. Unless they are in fruits, vegetables, whole grains, or engineered sports foods and drinks, simple carbohydrates in sweets are dispensable in a healthy diet.

## CHOOSE WHOLE GRAINS

The 2010 dietary guidelines recommend that at least half of grains consumed in a day come from whole grains. Studies show that consuming two to three servings of whole grains per day may reduce risk of cardiovascular disease, hypertension, diabetes, colon cancer, and obesity.[108] Make every attempt to consume at least three servings of whole grains per day. Each serving of whole grain should be about sixteen grams, for a total goal of forty-eight grams of whole grain per day.

High-fiber whole grains include whole-grain bread and pasta, brown rice, corn, and grains like quinoa, oats, bulgur, wheat, and barley. What is a whole grain? Whole grains contain the entire grain seed, called the kernel. There are three parts of the kernel: germ, bran, and endosperm. In contrast, refined grains have been processed to remove their bran and germ, leaving only the starchy endosperm. This process also removes fiber, iron, phytonutrients, and B vitamins. The enrichment process adds the B vitamins and iron back in refined grains.

The bran is the outer layer of the whole grain, rich in fiber, B vitamins, lignans, and trace minerals. The germ is the small, nutrient-rich core that contains antioxidants, vitamin E, B vitamins, and healthy fats, such as omega-3 fatty acids. The endosperm, occupying the majority of the grain, is the middle layer that contains carbohydrates and protein.

Fiber, also known as roughage or bulk, is the part of the food that the body cannot digest and break down. Plant foods like whole grains, fresh vegetables and fruits, beans, legumes, nuts, and seeds are all high in fiber. Fiber enhances the digestive system's transit time. In other words, fiber cleans the digestive tract to facilitate bowel movements and the removal of harmful substances, including cholesterol and carcinogens. Carcinogens are cancer-causing agents, many known to be in the foods we eat.

To be considered whole grain, a packaged product must have a minimum of 51 percent whole-grain ingredients by weight per serving. However, it is always best to exceed that minimum standard by seeking products that contain 100 percent whole grain. To be considered high fiber, the product must contain greater than 20 percent of the daily value.[109] Based on eating two thousand calories per day, a high-fiber food would contain four grams or more per serving on the food label.

Finding whole grains in packaged foods in the grocery store may be like walking through a labeling maze. With so many different terms on the food labels, distinguishing whole grains can be challenging—and just because the label says the product "contains whole grain" does not mean there is a sufficient amount of whole grain to make a healthful impact. The word *whole* should be listed first in the ingredient label in front of the specific grain. Look for terminology such as *whole-wheat flour*.

In your quest for whole-grain, high-fiber foods, another helpful tip is to utilize the rule of five. Search for healthy whole-grain products that have

five grams of fiber or more per serving;
five grams of protein or more per serving; and
fewer than five grams of sugars per serving.[110]

The Whole Grain Stamp on food packaging makes it much easier to find whole grains. Established by the not-for-profit Whole Grain Council, the yellow-and-brown Whole Grain Stamps help identify packaged foods containing whole grain. The Whole Grain Council also defines the standards the whole grain product must meet to be worthy of the stamp. Graphic 5.1 depicts the Whole Grain Stamps.[111]

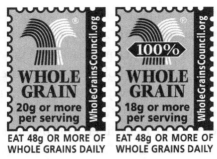

*Whole Grain Stamps are a trademark of Oldways Preservation Trust and the Whole Grains Council, www.wholegrainscouncil.org.*

There are two Whole Grain Stamps. The basic Whole Grain Stamp above means that there are eight grams of whole grain per serving but the product may also contain refined grains. The 100% Whole Grain Stamp means that there are sixteen grams of whole grain per serving with 100 percent of the grain ingredients coming from whole grain.[112]

Table 5.1 lists examples of whole grains. These should be listed first on the ingredient label to be considered whole grain. For example, barley is only whole grain when it has not been refined and would be listed as *whole-grain barley* on the ingredient label.

**Table 5.1: Examples of Whole Grains**

| | |
|---|---|
| Amaranth | Triticale |
| Teff | Rye |
| Barley | Buckwheat |
| Bulgur | Whole-grain corn |
| Millet | Whole-grain barley |
| Quinoa | Whole oats (e.g., steel-cut oats) |
| Sorghum | Whole wheat |
| Spelt | Wild, black, red, and brown rice |

Unfortunately, Americans eat too many refined grains listed in table 5.2 and not enough whole grains in table 5.1. Examples of refined grains include white or refined breads, cereals, and pasta. These refined grains are much lower in fiber and phytonutrients than whole grains. Certain foods with refined grains, such as cakes, cookies, and pies, are also high in sugar, calories, and saturated and trans fats—a nutritional train wreck.

**Table 5.2: Foods with Refined Carbohydrates**

| Cake, cookies, pie, gelatin, candy | Sugary beverages, fruit drinks, soda, energy drinks, sweetened tea |
|---|---|
| Pastries, muffins, doughnuts, pancakes | White rice |
| White bread, rolls, buns, bagels | Flour tortillas |
| Saltine crackers, snack chips, pretzels | Refined breakfast cereals |
| Pasta made with refined grains | Sugar, honey, agave, corn syrup, molasses, brown sugar |

The preference for refined carbs over whole grains (and fresh fruits and vegetables) causes the American diet to be low in fiber. According to the Institute of Medicine (IOM), American eaters get an average of fifteen grams of fiber per day. The IOM recommends getting fourteen grams of fiber for every one thousand calories consumed.[113] For most active adults, this would be in the range of twenty-five to thirty-five grams per day.

**Table 5.3: Fiber Intake Recommendations Based on Calories (Source: Institute of Medicine)**

| Calories Eaten Per Day | Fiber Per Day (g) |
|---|---|
| 1,500 | 21 |
| 1,800 | 25 |
| 2,000 | 28 |
| 2,500 | 35 |
| 3,000 | 42 |

Table 5.4 lists dietary fiber content of foods.[114]

**Table 5.4: Fiber Content of Foods (Source: USDA, Release 17)**

| | Fiber Content (g) |
|---|---|
| **Breads/Cereals/Grains** | |
| Whole Wheat Bread, 1 slice | 1.9 |
| Whole Wheat Pasta, 1 cup | 1.2 |
| All Bran, 3/4 cup | 13.2 |
| Raisin Bran Cereal, 3/4 cup | 5.5 |
| Cheerios, 3/4 cup | 2.7 |
| Brown Rice, 1 cup cooked | 3.6 |
| Corn Tortilla, 6 inch | 1 |
| **Legumes** | |
| Baked Beans, 1/3 cup canned | 3.4 |
| Black Beans, 1/2 cup canned | 7.5 |
| Kidney Beans, 1/2 cup canned | 8.2 |
| Garbanzo Beans, 1/2 cup canned | 5.3 |
| Lentils, 1/2 cup cooked | 7.8 |
| **Fruits** | |
| Apple, red w/ skin, medium | 3.3 |
| Banana, medium | 3.1 |

| | Fiber Content (g) |
|---|---|
| Blackberries, 1 cup | 7.6 |
| Blueberries, 1 cup | 3.5 |
| Raspberries, 1 cup | 8.0 |
| Strawberries, 1 cup | 3.3 |
| Figs, dried, 2 | 3.7 |
| Apricots, dried, 5 halves | 1.3 |
| Orange, fresh | 3.1 |
| **Vegetables** | |
| Broccoli, 1/2 cup raw | 1.2 |
| Corn, 1/2 cup cooked | 2.1 |
| Peas, green, 1/2 cup frozen | 4.4 |
| Potato, baked w/ skin | 5.5 |
| Sweet Potato, baked | 4.4 |
| **Nuts and Seeds** | |
| Almonds, 12 whole | 1.6 |
| Peanuts, roasted, 1 oz. | 2.3 |
| Sunflower seeds, 1 oz. | 2.6 |
| Chia seeds, 1 oz. | 10.6 |
| Flaxseeds, 1 oz. | 7.6 |

You can achieve the recommended twenty-five grams of fiber per day by replacing refined grains with foods containing whole grains as well as beans/legumes, nuts, seeds, and fresh fruits and vegetables. High-fiber packaged foods like whole-grain crackers, canned and dried beans, and trail mix identify their fiber content on the food label. Fiber is listed under the "Carbohydrates" section on the nutrition facts panel of the food label. If the food label touts a product to be "high fiber," it must contain three grams or more fiber per serving.

Be wary of foods with the "high fiber" designation that are

traditionally low in nutrition. Manufacturers are hopping on the fiber bandwagon by putting the "high fiber" designation on foods low in nutrition. These include everything from cookies to brownies to salty snack chips and sugary breakfast shakes. Get your fiber from whole foods—not high-sugar, salty, processed foods supplemented with fiber.

Take a new look at these high-fiber and nutrient-rich whole-grain favorites.

**Oats.** Although oats in the United States are commonly processed to produce "old-fashioned" or quick-cooking and instant oats, processed oats are among the few grains that still have their bran and germ intact. For those who still want a less-processed oat, steel-cut oats have become a popular whole-grain choice. Steel-cut oats are whole-grain groats cut into pieces. What's a groat? All types of oat cereal start as groats, which are hulled, toasted oat grains. The processing these groats undergo determines whether oats are rolled, instant, quick cooking, or steel cut.

Oatmeal is a delicious and nutritious way to get whole grains and soluble fiber. Replace low-fiber, sugary, neon-colored breakfast cereals with the goodness of oatmeal. A half cup of cooked oatmeal counts as a serving of whole grains. Look for oat and oat flour on the ingredient listing of foods containing oats. Traditional oatmeal can be nutritionally amped up with fresh or dried fruit, nuts, seeds, and cinnamon. Made with milk, including soy, rice, hemp, or almond milk, oatmeal becomes a meal in itself.

**Quinoa.** Did you ever associate a whole grain with being a worldwide trendsetter? Introducing quinoa. The Food and Agricultural Organization of the United Nations (FAO) recently declared 2013 to be recognized as the "International Year of Quinoa."[115] Quinoa (pronounced keen-wah) is popular from side dish to salad bar to main fare at gourmet restaurants. Quinoa is high in carbohydrates, protein, fiber, and the flavonoid antioxidants. The small amount of fat naturally found in quinoa contributes monounsaturated fats and the omega-3 fatty acid,

ALA. Quinoa has the distinction of containing all the essential amino acids to be a complete protein, very unusual for a plant-based source. Quinoa is versatile. It can be added to soups, salads, or pasta or served as a side dish. One half a cup of quinoa equals a serving of whole grain. Quinoa is gluten-free.

**Corn** is a whole grain. Relegating canned corn as a starchy side-plate vegetable is no longer the only way to serve corn. Popcorn, corn tortillas, fire-roasted corn, corn salsa and corn on the cob all count as servings of whole grain. Many varieties of corn tortilla chips combine their goodness with quinoa, black beans, and flax, sesame, and chia seeds. High in carbohydrates and fiber, corn is a popular and convenient choice to incorporate at the lunch or dinner table. Add corn to soups, stews, chili, tacos, and salads. Accompany these delicious foods with corn tortilla chips. Corn is gluten-free.

**Brown rice and wild rice** are superior over their processed white rice counterparts. Most restaurants now offer a brown rice option to their refined white rice mainstay. Use brown rice at home. Brown rice is as easy to prepare as white rice. Wild rice, actually a seed, is a healthy side dish or whole grain addition to soups and stuffing. Rice is gluten-free.

**Whole-grain breakfast cereals.** The highest fiber cereals will contain whole wheat, bran, brown rice, sorghum, and oats or a combination of these grains. The complex carbohydrates in whole-grain, high-fiber cereal fuel tennis longer than the rapid sugar rush attained from sugary, refined cereals. Whole-grain cereals that mix their nutrition with seeds (such as flax, pumpkin, and sunflower) are even more nutritious. Adding dried fruit (like raisins, apricots, and dates) boosts the fiber and nutritional content even further. Breakfast cereals are popular with children, teens, and adults. Make the most of one-third of your daily nutrition with a healthy whole-grain cereal, not a refined, sugary, artificially colored one.

# CARBS FUEL TENNIS

The most notable role of carbohydrates is their source of efficient energy or fuel for our working muscles. Carbs also fuel the brain, which is the only carbohydrate-dependent organ in our bodies. Fueling a car is a simplified analogy of how carbohydrates fuel our bodies. Your car needs gas to run. Moreover, your car needs the right type of gas to properly run. Would you put diesel fuel in a car that requires super unleaded? Surely not. Carbohydrates are the body's ideal fuel source.

Tennis involves brief periods of anaerobic, high-intensity effort, or bursts of energy, with periods of rest or low-intensity exercise. The immediate energy to chase down a lob or punch a volley is supplied by the hydrolysis of adenosine triphosphate, or ATP. ATP is a large molecule, stored in our cells in small amounts. When we exercise, we need to regenerate ATP as fast as it is used—to continue to contract muscles for those winning serves and ground strokes.

Regeneration of ATP requires an input of energy. There are three ways we obtain energy from ATP.[116] Listed below, each energy-production pathway has its specific use in athletic performance, including tennis. Many sports require and utilize a combination of all three pathways. Tennis makes use of the anaerobic pathways.

1. *Anaerobic: Breakdown of Creatine.* No oxygen is involved in regenerating ATP with anaerobic energy production. Hence, one way to generate ATP for quick energy is through the anaerobic means. Creatine phosphate is a natural substance found in our muscles. Our muscles contain 95 percent of the creatine in our bodies. During anaerobic activity, creatine phosphate donates its phosphate, which then binds with adenosine diphosphate (ADP), forming ATP. Although resynthesis of ATP through this

mechanism is very, very fast, it has low capacity, meaning fatigue can set in soon. This explains why this pathway is useful for athletic performance requiring quick, powerful bursts of energy, like sprints and weight lifting.

Creatine comes from protein-rich foods like meat and fish. Creatine is also a popular and readily available supplement. Creatine content in muscles can be increased by supplementing the diet. Creatine supplementation has been shown to enhance performance in athletics involving bursts of strength. (Refer to chapter 2 for more detail on creatine.)

2. *Anaerobic: Breakdown of Stored Glycogen to Lactate.* Like anaerobic use of creatine, the breakdown of stored glycogen in muscles is an anaerobic process, as well. However, its energy-producing pathway has its differences. Tennis play primarily draws on anaerobic breakdown of stored glycogen in muscle and liver, as well as triglycerides or fats in muscle and fat tissue. This pathway is a much slower energy-producing process than degradation of creatine but generates more energy and has unlimited capacity, as long as sufficient carbohydrates are consumed from food.

Glycogen is the storage form of glucose. Our muscles and liver store glycogen. Glycogen comes from carbohydrates in foods we eat. The process called glycolysis breaks down glycogen into glucose and then into the product called pyruvate. The body then converts pyruvate to lactate. For each pyruvate or glucose molecule converted to lactate, three ATP molecules form. Sustained intermittent exercise, like tennis, continues as glycolysis regenerates ATP.

Accumulation of lactate results in lactic acid buildup. This causes muscle pH to decrease and can have various effects on muscle, including fatigue. One popular yet unproven theory is that lactic acid accumulation causes both fatigue and muscle soreness, or "burn." We have all witnessed tennis players experiencing cramping on the court. This cramping can be a tennis player's most painful nightmare during a high-stakes match or tournament. Whether cramping is the result of lactic acid accumulation is still subject to recent debate. (Chapter 2 further discusses lactate production.)

3. ***Aerobic Energy Production.*** Unlike anaerobic activity, aerobic exercise, familiarly coined *cardio*, requires molecular oxygen to regenerate energy or ATP. In aerobic energy production, our bodies oxidize pyruvate generated from glucose to carbon dioxide and water. Continuous and sustained exercise, like medium- to long-distance running/jogging, swimming, cycling, and walking, relies on energy derived from the aerobic pathway. Producing ATP through the aerobic pathway is much slower than through anaerobic metabolism but generates considerably more energy and has unlimited capacity. This is because the fuel sources for aerobic production are both glycogen in the muscle and liver and triglycerides in muscle and fat tissue. Oxidation of just one glucose molecule in aerobic exercise results in 38 molecules of ATP production. Oxidation of one molecule of triglyceride or fat produces an astounding 127 molecules of ATP for energy. This explains how Boston marathon runners and Tour de France competitors are capable of sustaining their exercise output—through the practically unlimited fuel generated by the aerobic pathway.

Since aerobic exercise requires oxygen, the sustained power generated by aerobic energy production depends on our bodies' maximum rate of oxygen consumption. The maximum rate of oxygen consumption is called $VO_2$ max. $VO_2$ max is a measure of maximal aerobic capacity and varies greatly depending on age, sex, genetics, training, and health status. For example, a well-trained elite distance runner will have a significantly higher $VO_2$ max than his or her untrained counterpart. Males generally have a higher $VO_2$ max than females. Table 5.5 lists $VO_2$ max for typical activity groups.[117]

**Table 5.5: Typical $VO_2$ Max Values for Activity Groups (Source: *AND Sports Nutrition: A Practice Manual for Professionals*)**

| Activity Group | $VO_2$ max, range, ml/kg/min |
|---|---|
| Sedentary | 30–40 |
| Recreationally Active | 40–60 |
| Elite Endurance Athlete | 65–85 |

The above means of energy production do not operate independent of each other. Tennis may tap into the aerobic pathway for energy supply. Likewise, anaerobic energy production makes its contribution in a marathon race when energy demand is intermittently increased, like running up a hill, accelerating to pass a competitor, or sprinting to the finish line.

The production of ATP ultimately comes from the food substrates we eat. As this ideal source of food energy, carbohydrates play a vitally important role in energy production. Our bodies digest carbohydrates in foods containing sugars and starches and convert them to glucose, the simplest form of sugar. This digestion starts the minute that carbohydrates in food enter our mouths. Most of the starch breakdown occurs in the stomach and small intestine, where carbohydrates are further exposed to powerful enzymes from the pancreas and are reduced to simple sugar, or glucose, that then gets transported for use by our bodies.

Glucose travels throughout our bloodstream to fuel our muscles, brain, central nervous system, liver, and kidneys—organs and systems involved in athletic performance. Insulin, a hormone produced by the pancreas, pulls glucose from our blood into exercising muscles and the brain. Glucose is either oxidized, or "burned," as an immediate energy source or stored as glycogen in our muscles and liver for future use.

Glycogen is a long, complex chain of stored carbohydrate, readily available for fuel when needed. Liver glycogen stores maintain blood glucose levels at both rest and exercise. Muscle glycogen maintains blood glucose levels during exercise. We are constantly drawing from these liver and muscle glycogen stores all day and all night for energy—during sleep, during physical activity, and in between meals or fasting states.

At rest, like sleep, the brain utilizes most of the blood glucose while sedentary muscles use less than 20 percent of blood glucose. The liver is the source of glycogen at rest. During exercise, however, muscle glucose utilization can increase up to thirtyfold, depending on the duration and intensity of exercise. This prolific muscle utilization demonstrates the need for adequate carbohydrates for optimal athletic performance.

During intense exercise involving bursts of energy, characterized by tennis, our bodies primarily rely on glycogen, not triglycerides or fat, for energy. There is only a finite amount of glycogen available during intense exercise. The typical adult athlete stores about 1,800 calories worth of carbohydrate in the muscle, liver, and blood.

| A typical male stores the following amount of energy in his body: | | |
|---|---|---|
| Muscle glycogen = | 300–400 g or | 1,200–1,600 calories |
| Liver glycogen = | 75–100 g or | 300–400 calories |
| Blood glucose = | 25 g or | 100 calories |
| | | |
| Total Body Storage = | | 1,600–2,100 calories |

In general, about ten calories of glycogen are stored for every pound of body weight. A 120-pound woman stores about 1,200 calories worth of glycogen. A 190-pound man stores about 1,900 calories worth of glycogen. In contrast, the typical adult can store 100,000 calories in the form of body fat.

Remember, fat is not the ideal fuel source for muscles and the brain during anaerobic exercise. It is carbohydrates. Therefore, glycogen stores are the rate-limiting source of fuel during anaerobic exercise. We replenish these finite glycogen stores in our muscles and liver by eating more carbohydrates.

Glycogen stored in our muscles is used during exercise, while glycogen stored in the liver gets released into the bloodstream to maintain normal glucose levels in our blood. To reiterate, liver glycogen provides energy to the brain, although some is reserved for muscles. Muscle glycogen fuels exercise. Since we rely on our large muscles to play tennis, carbohydrates are essential in keeping our glycogen stores sufficient to fuel our powerful ground strokes, serves, and overheads.

The vital role carbohydrates play in performance is well studied in endurance sports, such as cycling, marathon running, and triathlons. Carbohydrates consumed before and during endurance sports have unquestionably demonstrated a delay in fatigue and enhancement in sports intensity and duration.[118] Marathon runners understand the importance of carbohydrate nutrition in their training preparation and in competition.

Research suggests that carbohydrates may also improve sports performance in intermittent stop-and-go sports, such as football, soccer, and tennis.[119] Since professional tennis has evolved into such a physically demanding sport, players must have the right fuel in the proper amounts for sustained power and high-intensity play from the start of the tennis match to the final winning point.

In his 2013 article in the *Journal of Sports Science and Medicine*, sports scientist Mayur Ranchordas and his team summarize practical nutrition recommendations for tennis. Ranchordas suggests elite tennis players follow a habitually high-carbohydrate diet of six to ten grams per kilogram of body weight per day. Elite tennis players train four hours or more per day. This amount is slightly less for women. For a 180-pound male, this would be 490–818 grams per day. For a 140-pound woman, this would be 381–636 grams, leaning toward the lower level of the range for elite women players.[120] This large amount of carbohydrate intake ensures adequate glycogen stores. This high number of calories also supports the training demands of competitive athletes whose calorie needs may be twice as high (or more) than the untrained athlete.

Although no studies have been done directly investigating glycogen concentrations during tennis, glycogen muscle depletion is a likely key cause of fatigue during tennis.[121] As we know very well, a singles tennis match can last a meager forty-five minutes or a grueling three hours. Carbohydrate planning ensures our bodies are well stocked with glycogen. Adequate glycogen stores ensure your body has the fuel to go the distance.

Carbohydrate planning is essential in tournament play when two or even three matches can be played over the course of a day. Tournament play usually involves travel, weather, or match delays and meal, rest, and even sleep disruptions. Since tournament day schedules can be irregular, having stored energy from carbohydrate planning is key to high-energy tennis performance.

## WHEN WE RUN OUT OF FUEL

Winning volleys, baseline rallies, and chasing down lobs can best happen when the body has a sufficient amount of glycogen stores. The amount of glycogen, or stored carbohydrate, is a limited resource. The amount of glycogen influences how long you can effectively play tennis, an important consideration when walking on the court or in a tournament, facing the unforeseen physical demands and duration of a match.

Unlike other sports that have defined time frames, such as

quarters in football, rounds in boxing, or periods in ice hockey, tennis has none, making it a mental and physical endurance sport in its own right. A most extreme example of this is the epic 2010 Wimbledon match between France's Nicolas Mahut and American John Isner. This extraordinary match, more than eleven hours long and played over two days, ended with a mind-boggling five set score of 6–4, 3–6, 6–7, 7–6, 70–68, the victory going to the valiant but spent Isner. The last set of this historic match lasted eight hours and eleven minutes!

When muscle and liver glycogen stores get too low, players "hit the wall." This unpleasant result of exhausted glycogen stores causes muscle fatigue, lack of stamina, poor athletic performance, and a mental yearning to quit—a nightmare that no tennis player ever wants to experience. I have talked with many tennis players who have experienced this augmented fatigue, particularly in matches they had not anticipated would go the distance. The lack of carbohydrate planning meant the difference between a win and a loss.

Liver glycogen maintains normal blood glucose levels to fuel our brain and muscles. When liver glycogen is depleted, another unpleasant phenomenon occurs, familiar in the running and cycling world as "bonking." Bonking is characterized by the feeling of dizziness or light-headedness, irritability, and lack of focus and coordination. This occurs because the liver is not releasing enough stored carbohydrate or sugar into the bloodstream.[122] Bonking is analogous to having low blood sugar during tennis. Keep in mind that while muscles can store glycogen, the brain cannot. Thus, carbohydrates must be consumed shortly before exercise—that big tennis match—to immediately supply a source of glucose or fuel to the brain.

Bonking can be brought to life in a common tennis scenario. When we skip our breakfast before a tennis match after fasting all night and do not eat or drink foods or fluids with carbohydrates, we can experience symptoms like sweating, dizziness, shakiness, weakness, and blurred vision. The resultant low blood glucose is detrimental to any sports activity—most importantly, it is dangerous.

Fortunately, fast-acting carbohydrates, such as sports gels, juice, and sports drinks provide the immediate remedy for low blood glucose levels. Always follow this quick fix for low blood sugar with an easily digestible small meal with protein—a sandwich or yogurt smoothie are good options. This ensures your blood glucose levels normalize, as well as your tennis performance. Winning tennis depends on well-fueled muscles and a well-fueled brain.

## THE GLYCEMIC INDEX

Sports gels, sports drinks, rice cakes, and pretzels are a few examples of carbohydrate-containing foods having a high glycemic index. Glycemic index (GI) is the measure of how quickly blood sugar levels rise after eating a carbohydrate-containing food.[123] A food with a higher GI raises blood sugar more quickly than a food with a lower GI.

Right before a match, food and drink with a high GI provide quick energy to fuel the brain—a half cup of a sports drink, a handful of sports beans, or a couple of rice cakes will provide fast-acting carbohydrates. In contrast, complex carbohydrates in many starchy foods like beans, whole grains, and starchy fruits and vegetables tend to have a lower GI and may be most effective when eaten well before a match to promote glycogen storage and a steady, sustained release of sugar.

Low GI foods, such as beans, whole-grain bread, and peas are also high in fiber and can be difficult to digest, causing gas. Therefore, they are not the most digestible—hence, desirable— sources of carbohydrate right before a tennis match. Save the beans and brown rice hours before or a day or two before your big match when your body has time to digest this healthy, high-fiber meal. No tennis match can be played well with a gassy or bloated digestive tract. Table 5.6 lists low, medium and high GI foods.[124]

**Table 5.6: GI of Foods, American Diabetes Association, 2014**

| Low GI Foods (GI = 55 or less) |
| --- |
| Oatmeal (steel-cut or rolled), muesli, oat bran |
| 100 percent stone-ground whole-wheat or pumpernickel bread |
| Pasta, converted rice, barley, bulgur |
| Sweet potato, corn, legumes, lentils, peas |
| Most fruits, nonstarchy vegetables, and carrots |
| **Medium GI Foods (GI = 56–69)** |
| Whole-wheat, rye, and pita bread |
| Quick-cooking oats |
| Brown, wild, or basmati rice, couscous |
| **High GI Foods (GI = 70 or more)** |
| White bread or bagel |
| Corn flakes, puffed rice, instant oatmeal, bran flakes |
| Short-grain white rice |
| Russet potato, pumpkin |
| Pretzels, rice cakes, popcorn, saltine crackers |
| Melons and pineapple |

Many factors influence the GI of foods. Since tennis players frequently toss a trusty banana in their tennis bags, its GI is worthy of discussion. Ripeness of fruit will influence its GI. A ripe banana that has a higher sugar content than a green, unripe banana will have a higher GI. Be sure to pack a palatable, ripe banana in your tennis bag for its valuable starch and sugar content. How food is processed also influences GI. Juice has a higher GI than the whole fruit with skin. Mashed potatoes have a higher GI than a baked potato with the skin.[125]

The GI value represents the type of carbohydrate in a food and the rate it raises blood sugar. As its nomenclature indicates, it is an index. The GI of a food does not take into account portion sizes, which will influence the total amount of carbohydrate consumed.

## CARBS: HOW MUCH, WHEN, AND WHY?

How much carbohydrate should a tennis player consume? The answer depends on a number of variables that need to be thought of ahead of time.

1. **Exercise intensity.** Are you playing singles or doubles tennis? Singles play requires far more physical stamina than doubles, obviously due to the greater energy output required for singles compared to doubles play. If you are competing in a singles tennis match, having adequate glycogen stores becomes especially important.

2. **Exercise type.** Carbohydrate timing varies with exercise type. Resistance and endurance training require a different nutrition prescription than tennis does. As their intensity level and duration are different, so too would their sports nutrition regimen.

3. **Weight.** How much do you weigh? Carbohydrate (as well as protein and fat) ingestion is dependent on total calories, which is influenced by weight.

4. **Exercise duration.** Are you playing a singles match in one day or a more demanding two or three matches over a tournament day? As expected, increased glycogen stores are necessary for tennis on tournament day, when endurance becomes an important performance consideration.

5. **Age.** Are you an adult, teen, or child?

6. **Trained or untrained.** How well trained are your muscles? Untrained muscles are not nearly as efficient in storing glycogen compared to trained muscles. Athletes who are well trained can store significantly more glycogen than untrained athletes.

The International Society for Sports Nutrition (ISSN) suggests that athletes consume 65 percent of calories from carbohydrates and then a slightly higher rate of 70 percent of calories five to seven days prior to competition to maximize muscle and liver storage of glycogen.[126] Nonathletes should consume about 55 percent of total calories from carbohydrates. Each gram of carbohydrate contains four calories. Using two thousand calories as a typical day's total caloric intake for a nonathlete, the amount of carbohydrates are calculated as follows:

2,000 calories/day × 55 percent of calories from carbohydrate per day (0.55) = 1,100 calories from carbohydrates

1,100 calories from carbohydrate ÷ 4 calories per gram of carbohydrate = 275 grams carbohydrate/day

Elite competitive tennis players who undergo intense training may need twice as many calories, upward of three thousand to five thousand calories per day. Therefore, the carbohydrate need will be doubled too. Similarly, nonathletes may need fewer than two thousand calories per day. An RD or CSSD can help determine your calorie needs based on your physical activity level, training, and other needs unique to you.

Other sports scientists suggest basing carbohydrate guidelines on weight to account for the person's size and muscle mass. This method may correlate better to fuel requirements and actual consumption compared to calculating carbohydrate based on a percentage of contribution to total daily energy intake. Carbohydrate needs based on mass are individualized to an athlete's training or competition demands. This also provides more practical carbohydrate targets in situations where calorie needs are extremely high (e.g., four thousand to five thousand calories per day).

Experts recommend athletes with light training schedules should consume three to five grams per kilogram of body weight per day. Athletes with moderate-intensity training for sixty minutes a day should consume five to seven grams per kilogram of body weight per day. Athletes engaged in moderate- to high-intensity endurance exercise lasting one to three hours per day should consume upward of six to ten grams per kilogram of body weight per day.[127] Six to ten grams per kilogram of body weight per day concurs with the suggested carbohydrate intake from Ranchordas in his review of nutrition practice guidelines for elite tennis players.[128]

These recommendations represent the following daily carbohydrate intake in a person who weighs 150 pounds:

| | |
|---|---|
| Light training | 205–340 g carbohydrate/day |
| Moderate training | 340–477 g carbohydrate/day |
| High-intensity endurance training | 409–680 g carbohydrate/day |

To put this amount in perspective, a slice of bread, a small piece of fruit, or a half cup of cooked oatmeal contains about fifteen grams of carbohydrate. One may think that a figure like 340 grams of carbohydrate per day is an insurmountable amount to consume. But look how this simple, modest breakfast meal adds up in needed carbohydrates:

| | |
|---|---|
| 1/2 cup orange juice | 15 g carbohydrate |
| 1 cup unsweetened dry cereal | 30 g carbohydrate |
| 1 medium banana | 20 g carbohydrate |
| 1/2 cup skim or soy milk | 6 g carbohydrate |
| Total carbohydrates = | 71 g |

Seventy-one grams is approximately 21 percent of the 340 grams of carbohydrate per day—in one nutrient-packed, easy-to-prepare breakfast meal.

Well-planned carbohydrates prior to and during match play are essential for athletic performance. Singles tennis play is more physically demanding than doubles play. Adding the demands of an all-day tournament with a minimum of two matches per day plus practice sessions make carbohydrate nutrition essential for tennis stamina and endurance. Plan and time carbohydrates around your activity. Playing singles in a tournament would make meal planning more critically important compared to a casual Sunday morning doubles match.

The International Tennis Foundation (ITF) Coach Education Series provides excellent advice on nutrition for tennis players.[129] These tips encourage carbohydrates at all stages of match play: before, during, and after. (Look for more detail on menu ideas for nutrient timing in chapter 11.)

**Table 5.7: Carbohydrate and Meal Planning for Tennis Players (Source: ITF)**

| Prematch | Eating Tips |
| --- | --- |
| Two days preceding match | Increase carbohydrate intake to ensure glycogen stores are high. This can be accomplished by consuming 55–65 percent of calories from carbs (refer to above example) throughout the day. |
| Night before a match | Continue to consume carbohydrate and lean protein in meals. Good examples include pasta with sauce, fish and rice, or poultry with baked potato—all with salad and/or vegetables and fresh fruit. Choose light desserts like frozen yogurt, fruit, oatmeal cookie. |

| Match Day | |
|---|---|
| Morning match | Eat a light, high-carb breakfast, such as cereal with low-fat milk, whole-grain toast with lightly spread peanut butter, or oatmeal with dried or fresh fruit. |
| Midday match | In addition to breakfast, have an easy-to-digest midmorning snack, like fresh fruit, granola bar, fruit/yogurt smoothie, pretzels. |
| Afternoon match | For lunch, carbohydrate and lean protein, such as turkey or tuna fish sandwich, with fresh fruit or salad or lean hamburger on a bun w/ lettuce, tomato, and fruit. *Avoid greasy, hard-to-digest fried foods (like french fries, nachos and cheese, hot dogs).* |
| **Postmatch** | |
| | Eat a healthy, high-carbohydrate meal with protein and fat to restore glycogen; nourish, repair, and rebuild muscles; and replenish calories for energy. Good examples include tofu, fish, chicken, or lean beef with baked sweet potato or rice and vegetables. Replenishing calories through dessert is fine as long as postmatch nutrient needs are met first. |

It was thought that the amount of carbohydrate used by our bodies reached a ceiling of one gram per minute, meaning that the most carbohydrate from food and fluids our bodies could absorb and effectively use during activity was sixty grams in an hour. There are sixty grams of carbohydrate in twenty-four ounces of sports drink. Recent studies show that multiple sources of carbohydrate during exercise can exceed this limit, making the delivery and utilization of glucose fuel by muscles higher than was once thought.[130]

Studies repeatedly show that a mixture of carbohydrate sources in proper amounts can decrease perceived exertion, decrease fatigue, enhance performance, and improve power output.[131] Carbohydrates during exercise should consist of a mixture of glucose, maltodextrin, and fructose. A medium banana and sixteen ounces of sports drink consumed during each hour of exercise provides sixty grams of carbohydrates through multiple sugars to enhance transport, delivery, and utilization by working tennis muscles. (Chapter 8 provides further examples of carbohydrate-containing snacks that can best fuel tennis.)

## THE LOW-CARB DIET IS A TENNIS FOE

Depriving the body of carbohydrates on low-carb, high-protein diets causes the body to use protein and fat for energy—which are not ideal fuel sources. Remember the analogy of using the best fuel source for your car? Protein and fat are not as effective fuel sources when compared to carbohydrates.

Protein and fat have more vital roles, such as building new muscle, healing, and providing essential fatty acids and fat-soluble vitamins. Only 50 percent of protein turns into glucose in the blood. Only 10 percent of fat turns into glucose. Although these nutrients have important roles, they are not the primary energy source we draw from during the anaerobic exercise demands of tennis.

Protein and fat cannot effectively perform their primary functions if they are used as a calorie or fuel source when the body is deprived of carbohydrates. Despite what you may hear, making ketones, a waste product of using fat for energy, is not good for you and is physiologically stressful on our kidneys.

Many folks ask, "Then why do I lose so much weight when I eliminate carbs from my diet?" Any diet that is lower in calories than the body needs to maintain its weight will make you lose weight. Pure fact: excess calories, not carbohydrates, in our diet are "fattening."

Because carbohydrates should contribute up to 55–65 percent of your daily caloric intake, even higher for athletic performance, eliminating them on a low- or no-carb diet could cause you to eliminate over half your calories! For example, if you eat two thousand calories a day and eliminate carbs and do not replace them with other calories, you could be eliminating one thousand calories a day. You would be subsisting on a mere one thousand calories—inadequate to provide the energy and nutrients your tennis body needs.

These low-carb and gimmicky diets make you lose weight. They might be packaged and marketed as the new diet on the block, when the fundamental reason these diets cause weight loss is through a steep caloric reduction—often an unhealthy, drastic one at that. The next time you consider a low-carb or weight-loss diet, ask yourself this critical question: "Can I follow this diet for the rest of my life?" Chances are, the answer will be a firm no.

This definitely applied to Andrew, the teaching pro introduced in the beginning of the chapter. He quickly fatigued from his rigid low-carb-diet regimen consisting of chicken breast and vegetables. He learned that excess total calories cause weight gain, not carbs, gladly adding the proper amount of healthy carb-containing foods back into his tennis diet. He enjoyed eating again and had a much higher energy level to fuel his busy tennis lifestyle.

# 6

# WINNING THE GAME OF WEIGHT MANAGEMENT

**If you don't take care of your body,
where are you going to live?**
—Unknown

Donna has always wanted to lose that pesky fifteen pounds of extra weight—to play better and look better. She bought herself new stylish tennis outfits one size smaller to inspire her weight-loss effort. Like many of her friends at the tennis club, Donna has tried a number of diets, from the cabbage soup diet to the Paleo diet to vitamin-infused weight-loss shakes—she has lost track of the many ways she has lost and then regained weight in her yo-yo dieting. Despite dropping weight on these calorie-restrictive diets, she admits feeling fatigued, not to mention missing her favorite foods. She starts eating more to fulfill her hunger and appetite cravings. Her long-term weight management success falls short of her ever believing she can fit into her new tennis outfits. At this point, Donna would be happy to lose five pounds—if only she could keep it off for good.

Tennis players need to be physically fit to be on top of their game. This means not only achieving an ideal weight but also attaining peak fitness level. Excellent footwork, flexibility, strength, quickness, and endurance happen when the tennis player is physically fit. Nutrition is a key component of the physical conditioning necessary for optimal tennis performance.

Steve Smith is a brilliant junior tennis coach and developer in Tampa, Florida. He has fostered the junior development of hundreds of elite collegiate and professional tennis players. He is founder of Tennissmith, a resource and service dedicated to teaching tennis to the highest level of competency. I interviewed Smith to gain his thoughtful insights on the state of American youth tennis and how diet is taking its toll on the fitness levels of our future players. Smith goes so far as to say that today's fitness trainer is as important as his or her tennis coach.[132] Peak fitness in competitive tennis pays great dividends. The player who moves more quickly and lasts longer will be the winner.

The difference between being in the top one hundred in the tennis profession compared to the top ten can legitimately be attributed to physical fitness level. The same can be applied to all tennis arenas, whether it be the club, collegiate, or professional level. Professional tennis players who have dramatically improved their nutrition and physical conditioning, catapulting to number one in the world, include Martina Navratilova, Ivan Lendl, Andre Agassi, and Novak Djokovic to name a few. Djokovic, the extremely fit Serbian phenom, has attributed his tennis success in substantial part to a gluten-free diet and physical conditioning.

Scottish star Andy Murray and American Mardy Fish are two other professional players who, with weight loss and physical conditioning, shook up the professional rankings. Like his competitive nemesis Novak Djokovic, Murray underwent a physical transformation, diet included, to win his first Grand Slam title at the US Open in 2012. He went on to win the gold medal in the 2012 summer Olympics. He became the hometown hero, winning the coveted Wimbledon title in 2013—his lifelong dream fulfilled.

After a near-career-ending knee surgery in 2009, Mardy Fish lost thirty pounds and reduced his body fat from 21 percent to a modest 7 percent. He transformed his body and his game. Fish had his most successful year, entering the 2010 US Open as the ATP's number-one seed for the American men. In the August 31, 2010, *New York Times* feature "Fish Drops Weight and Adds Wins," reporter Harvey Araton summarizes Fish's thoughts on his first round US Open win: "Not to brag," but Fish said he "not only felt fine as the 2 hour and 36 minute match progressed, but the weather was nothing to sweat about either." This came from the American veteran who used to "tire quickly, really quickly."

Excellent footwork, quickness, and endurance happen when the tennis player is at both an ideal weight and fitness level. However, losing weight is distinctly different from getting fit. Fitness training can include weight loss as part of the conditioning process. Improving fitness level also includes many other facets. Working on key tennis elements, such as balance, agility, flexibility, endurance, and muscular strength, should be included in a tennis fitness program. Being thin does not equate to fitness, and being overweight does not mean that one is unfit. A certified athletic trainer (ATC) or certified personal trainer (CPT) can provide the assistance needed to manage weight and improve fitness level. A CSSD or RD can teach you how to get the right nutrition for tennis-specific weight management.

The challenge in getting into top physical conditioning results from cultural culprits promoting an overweight, unfit society. The cause of an overweight, unfit society is poor diet and sedentary activity level. Overweight and obesity are two of the end results, among many other consequential health outcomes. Two-thirds of Americans are either overweight or obese. This statistic is alarming. If you fall into this category, make a concerted effort to manage weight not only for improved tennis fitness but for lifelong health.

Obesity is a risk factor for a multitude of chronic diseases, including hypertension or high blood pressure, heart disease, and diabetes. Obesity is also a risk factor for joint disease, gallstones, sleep apnea, and other respiratory or breathing conditions. Obesity adversely affects quality of life. The Center for Disease Control and Prevention (CDC) reports that in 2008, addressing obesity and its related chronic illnesses resulted in a staggering $147 billion in health care costs, with half of that amount being paid by Medicare and Medicaid dollars.[133]

The weight-loss industry has responded. In dealing with this overweight and obesity epidemic, it has become a $35 billion business. The likelihood of these dollars augmenting, both in health care cost and the weight-loss industry, is palpable. Obesity in America is truly a plague gone out of control.

Overweight and obesity are defined by body mass index, or BMI. BMI is a ratio of weight to body surface area. BMI is calculated from your weight and your height. A BMI less than 18.5 classifies a person as being underweight. BMI of 18.5–24.9 is within normal limits. BMI between 25 and 29.9 means a person is overweight. A BMI of 30 or greater classifies a person as obese.[134] It is important to know your BMI. The below websites provide reliable BMI calculators: nhlbisupport.com/bmi/bmiinojs.htm and cdc.gov/healthyweight /assessing/index.html.

Below are the classification guidelines for weight status using BMI.

**Table 6.1: BMI Levels (Source: World Health Organization)**

| Weight Status | BMI (kg/m2) |
|---|---|
| Underweight | <18.5 |
| Normal Weight | 18.5–24.9 |
| Overweight | 25–29.9 |
| Obesity (Class 1) | 30–34.9 |
| Morbid Obesity (Class 2) | 35–39.9 |
| Class 3 | 40 or greater |

Weight gain occurs when the body takes in more calories than it needs. When the body cannot oxidize, or "burn," them through physical activity, this imbalance causes excess calories to be stored. In contrast, weight loss occurs when there is a reduction in calories consumed and/or an increase in caloric expenditure through physical activity. Theories on obesity abound, but the bottom line is this caloric imbalance is what causes overweight and obesity.

Americans need to discern two distinct terms: weight loss versus weight management. Weight loss occurs by restricting calories, increasing calories expended through physical activity, or both. Weight management is keeping weight at its healthiest throughout the life span through physical activity and healthy eating habits.

Weight loss tends to be transient characterized by the common scenario of diet followed / diet stopped / weight regained, a.k.a. yo-yo dieting. Weight management, on the other hand, is a lifelong process. People who are most successful at achieving and maintaining a healthy weight do so through the disciplined consumption of calories from foods and beverages to meet their energy needs while being physically active.

Women who restrict calories should consume no fewer than 1,200 calories per day. Men should consume no fewer than 1,500 calories per day. Nutritional needs are very difficult to meet or cannot be met at caloric levels lower than these parameters, unless vitamin and mineral supplements are taken. Severe caloric restrictions may provide the immediate gratification of quick weight loss but seldom lead to long-term weight management.

For athletes, this subpar caloric intake cannot fuel peak tennis performance. Competitive tennis players with rigorous training schedules may need two to three times the calories listed above. For elite athletes wanting to lose weight, calorie levels need to be adequate to support athletic performance. Working with an ACT and a CSSD or RD for specific fitness training and dietary guidance can help manage weight while sustaining athletic performance.

Cutting calories in the absence of exercise causes muscle and water loss. Since muscle is more metabolically active than fat tissue, the muscle lost through dieting results in a less efficient metabolism. This is the reason why overly restrictive fad diets fail.

Most trendy "diets of the month" can be very low in calories as well as nutrition. Be wary of diets whose calorie levels have triple digits, because there is no way they can provide the nutrition your active tennis body needs in such limited volumes of food or fluids without supplementation. Weight loss can easily occur on unhealthy, even dangerous, diets providing only six hundred or seven hundred calories per day, barely enough for sustenance. However, you will feel this caloric and nutrient deprivation on the tennis courts through fatigue, weakness, and lack of motivation—absolute pitfalls to tennis performance.

Calories provide the energy required by our bodies to carry out its many life functions. Calories are necessary; excessive calories are not. Energy is expended or burned by metabolism, or utilization of the calories in the food we eat. When we eat the same number of calories from food as we oxidize, or burn, we maintain weight in homeostatic balance.

Homeostasis is the body's drive to balance itself at a certain weight or "set point." Despite the alarming overweight and obesity statistics, our bodies' homeostasis maintains a very narrow weight margin: surprisingly, our weight is adaptively set to remain steady. Calories consumed equal calories or energy expended. Then what has caused America's weight to go so awry? When cultural components affect this physiologic equilibrium, including high-calorie diets, rushed eating, and sedentary lifestyle, caloric imbalance results. This can be better explored by understanding the components of energy expenditure.

## COMPONENTS OF ENERGY EXPENDITURE

There are three components of energy expenditure:

1. **Resting energy expenditure (REE)** is the energy burned in the activities necessary to sustain normal bodily functions, including breathing, circulation, making new cells, and maintenance of body temperature. These are the calories needed to sustain life. Factors that affect REE include the following:[135]

   a. **Body composition.** The major single determinant of REE is the amount of lean mass or muscle compared to fat in our bodies. This is referred to as our body composition. Muscle is far more metabolically active than fat. Metabolism is defined as the rate at which we burn calories. This means muscle burns calories more efficiently than fat. If you recall, muscle is gained and preserved through exercise and resistance training.

   b. **Body size.** Larger people have a higher REE than smaller statured people. A large tennis player with a formidable stature of six foot five and 220 pounds would require hundreds, even thousands, of more calories compared to a petite tennis player half this size.

   c. **Gender.** Since men have a greater proportion of muscle mass compared to women, they have higher rates of REE.

   d. **Age.** As we age, body size and composition change, most notably the loss of lean muscle mass. Our REE declines approximately 2–3 percent per every decade we age after early adulthood. While 2–3 percent sounds like a drop in the bucket, when added up, this can be significant pounds of weight gain over time.

      Just think, from the age of thirty to fifty, assuming

our metabolism slows by 6 percent (3 percent per decade), we would need to consume 6 percent fewer calories or expend that much more energy each day to maintain our weight. If you are used to eating 2,000 calories per day when you were thirty, by the time you are fifty, you would need to eat 120 calories fewer per day, or eat the same but burn 120 calories more per day. Sounds so simple, but in reality, we have made it a daunting task. Many of us do the opposite and actually eat more and expend less energy in our older years. An extra 120 calories not utilized each day equates to 12.5 pounds of extra weight in one year!

There are other factors influencing REE. Fever significantly increases the body's metabolism or the rate at which we burn energy. Remember the expression "Starve a cold; feed a fever"? Truth lies in this adage, because we quickly burn calories with the presence of fever. Athletes also have a higher REE. A muscularly lean athlete will have an efficient metabolism. Athletes like runners or triathletes with single-digit body fat percentage are like calorie-burning furnaces.

2. **Thermic Effect of Food.** Our bodies actually burn calories when we eat. This is known as the thermic effect of food. We utilize energy to digest and absorb food. Thermic effect of food accounts for about 10 percent of total energy expenditure. Spicy foods and caffeine actually stimulate the thermic effect of food.

3. **Physical Activity.** This is the most variable determinant of total energy expenditure or calories burned. An individual who is a sedentary couch potato would require far fewer calories than a physically active singles tennis player who may require twice as many (or more) calories through training and competition. Physical activity causes muscles to burn carbohydrates, protein, and fat for energy.

Notice the recurring theme on energy expenditure. The higher proportion of lean muscle to adipose (fat) tissue gained through physical activity will make you more efficient in burning calories from food. Combine regular physical activity with healthy food choices for a surefire way to successfully manage weight.

The versatility of tennis provides the option of singles or doubles play. Each type of play delivers very different physical demands. As much as casual doubles tennis is wonderful recreation, the amount of physical activity is limited. Casual doubles tennis players who need to lose weight (or not) should supplement their tennis game with cardiovascular fitness training and diet management. Always seek the advice of a health professional before engaging in a cardiovascular program for weight management, especially if you are elderly and/or have conditions that necessitate medical attention.

## THE REAL REASONS WHY DIETS DON'T WORK

You have heard it over and over: diets do not work. There is science behind this statement. Restrictive diets deprive. This deprivation has distinct consequences on our brain and body. When we consume a diet very low in calories, the body goes in an adaptive semistarvation mode. Sensing the decline in calories, the stomach comes to the rescue by releasing the hormone ghrelin. Ghrelin signals the brain to produce further chemicals that stimulate the appetite—in other words, make us want to eat—when we are dieting.

It is no wonder why folks on hypocaloric diets crave the foods they love and often have bigger appetites. They may think it is "in their head," beating themselves up in their spiral of downward deprivation, when, in fact, there is a physiological basis behind bigger cravings and bigger appetites on restrictive diets.

In contrast, when we eat and our stomach feels full, our bodies release hormones that tell our brain we are full. Fat cells release the hormone leptin, which signals the brain we are satiated. The brain then releases chemicals to suppress appetite and stop eating. Without leptin to make us feel full, we would eat incessantly or gorge. This neurohormonal signaling takes several minutes and explains why quickly scarfing down a large meal can make us feel uncomfortably full before leptin can do its job in telling the brain we are satiated—the science behind the words of wisdom to take twenty minutes or longer to eat a meal.

Taking the time to eat, savor, and enjoy meals is important. This allows time for your brain to receive hormonal signals that your hunger is satisfied. Another recently discovered hormone, peptide YY, also signals the brain to suppress appetite after eating. Bariatricians are medical doctors who specialize in treating obesity and related disorders. Among other laboratory analysis, they can determine if this neurohormonal response regulating hunger and appetite is normal.

A parallel physiological response happens when we eat foods we find especially tasty. When we eat sugar-, fat-, and salt-laden foods (or what we deem as pleasurable foods), the brain releases "pleasure" neurotransmitters, or brain chemicals, such as endorphin, dopamine, norepinephrine, and serotonin. Many activities motivate us to want to feel good, like eating delicious, palatable foods that restrictive diets eliminate.

Food gets us excited and gives us pleasure. The neurotransmitters dopamine, serotonin, and norepinephrine are associated with food seeking, appetite, and mood. The desire for pleasure is a result of a normal response by the brain and therefore explains why we crave the foods we have been deprived of. We want to satisfy this hedonistic need, not just our hunger. Diets challenge our bodies and brains' normal physiology. They work against us, not with us.

So, how does one manage weight without being caught in the vortex of trendy, even unsafe diets of the month? First, change your perspective about food. Rather than focusing on eliminating foods or entire food groups from your diet, include all foods in moderation.

Moderation sounds mundane and uninspiring. However, it works. Moderation means balancing healthy foods with occasional "empty calories," while keeping portions in control. Moderation is the timeless approach to eating healthily and managing weight. Moderation requires attention, focus, and discipline. Moderation puts the accountability back on the individual—not on the latest diet fad. Moderation is about inclusion, not exclusion.

The fat-free and low-fat diets in the '80s and '90s are a good example of how exclusion of food groups does not lead to weight-management success. When the public was excluding fat from their diets through fat-free and low-fat versions of almost every imaginable processed food, Americans became more overweight than ever. Those calories from vilified fat were replaced mostly with calories from carbohydrates, particularly simple sugars. Low fat or fat-free does not necessarily equate to low calorie. Like disco and shoulder pads, fat-free and very-low-fat diets went out with the era. The elimination of an entire macronutrient—fat in foods containing fat—does not result in long-term weight loss or health promotion when those calories are replaced with unhealthy foods.

Carbohydrates, protein, and fat are essential nutrients that need to be in proper balance. As a registered dietitian, I have worked with many individuals in their quest to lose weight. For some, this has been a lifelong challenge. The following are common real-life challenges from those who have been both successful and unsuccessful in their weight management attempts.

## WEIGHT MANAGEMENT SCENARIO #1: THE EMOTIONAL EATER

We have all eaten in response to our emotional state rather than in response to hunger. However, many of us are consistently unable to find the proper balance between emotional eating and mindful eating. Over time, this caloric imbalance may lead to challenges in managing weight unless the underlying reasons for overeating are addressed. Mindful eating is based on hunger cues as opposed to the emotional aspects of appetite. Depression, anxiety, stress, guilt, and boredom may cause us to eat more (or fewer) calories than required.

Are you thinking about trying another diet to lose weight? Before you do, understand the concept of mindful eating first— and it may forever change the way you view eating. Diets focus on what we eat, whereas mindful eating addresses why we eat to begin with.

In her best-selling book *Am I Hungry? What to Do When Diets Don't Work*, Michelle May, MD, discusses the "eat-repeat-repent" cycle frequently associated with emotional eating versus mindful eating. May believes that in order to successfully manage weight, the reasons we eat need to be explored and addressed.[136]

Hunger is the need to eat; appetite is the desire to eat. Hunger is the body's physiological signal telling us we need food. Hunger, like thirst, cannot be controlled or ignored; it is instinctive. Prolonged hunger can lead to dizziness, fatigue, and lack of focus—enemies on the tennis court.

Appetite is more complicated than hunger. Appetite occurs through a coordinated effort between the brain and the stomach. Appetite is a learned response to properties of food, such as taste, texture, and aroma. Ever go to the movies and eat buttered popcorn, loads of it, even when you are not hungry? Hot dogs, beer, and cotton candy at a baseball game? Nachos, pizza, and beer at a Super Bowl party? The list goes on. This type of eating is an example of learned response. Many moviegoers cannot resist the aroma and thought of munching on warm, fresh popcorn—even when they are not hungry—causing them to eat excessive calories. Similarly, pleasure emotions evoke appetite. Just the mere thought or smell of food can elicit appetite.

Unlike hunger, appetite can be ignored—not always an easy endeavor when these behaviors have been learned throughout a lifetime of individualized cues. To address emotional eating, hunger and appetite need to be distinguished. Condition yourself to eat when you are hungry. If only this could be so simple.

Eating in response to hunger tends to be very challenging for many who struggle with weight. The next time you think about eating, stop and ask yourself, "Am I hungry?" If not, can your appetite be distracted by means other than food, such as reading, taking a walk, or playing tennis? Becoming aware of these emotional triggers allows you to take action to address them without food.

In her book *Am I Hungry? What to Do When Diets Don't Work*, May describes three types of eaters: those out of control, those in control, and those in charge. People out of control are overeaters. Their hunger cues are completely misaligned with their eating behavior. They eat for many reasons besides being hungry (stress, boredom, depression, anxiety) and thereby end up overeating.[137]

People in control of their eating may appear focused and disciplined. However, they still use many emotional cues to eat (or not eat). For example, they may eat based on what the clock dictates or by rituals rather than because of hunger.[138] At its most extreme, these behaviors can result in anorexia nervosa—an eating disorder characterized by excessive control over eating, which requires professional attention.

People in charge of their eating eat when they are hungry. They have the healthiest relationship with food.[139] If you know your eating is due to reasons other than hunger, take charge and focus on instinctive eating—by doing so, resorting to the next weight-loss diet may be a thing of the past.

Another foremost expert on the topic of mindful eating is Dr. Susan Albers. Albers is a psychologist who specializes in mindful eating, weight loss, and body image concerns. She has written five books, including *Eating Mindfully*. She shares her information and insights on her website: www.eatingmindfully. com. Albers's mindful eating plate provides the tenets of the mindful philosophy: being aware, eating in the moment with no distractions, savoring food, and being nonjudgmental about your eating behaviors and attitudes.[140]

I recall working with a young gentleman named Danny. Danny was a successful salesman in his midthirties who desperately wanted to lose weight. The extra fifteen pounds he wanted to drop felt like an unattainable fifty pounds. The struggle with his weight and body image took a toll on his mental health too. After work, he would go home and watch hours of television while dozing or napping. The only thing that made him feel good was eating his favorite comfort foods, like chips, chicken wings, and ice cream, almost always alone on the couch or in bed in front of the television. He slept a lot. He dared not go to the gym or socialize with friends. How could he expose his out-of-shape body and shameful eating habits to anyone? He felt he was a failure, incapable of dropping a mere fifteen pounds. Turns out, Danny was depressed. His altered body image was a result of clinical depression. Once he got professional help, he was able to refocus on behaviors to positively manage his weight.

## EATING DISORDERS

More serious, disordered eating can manifest itself through binge eating, bulimia, and anorexia nervosa. The most notable tennis player who has candidly shared her struggles with her weight and binge eating disorder is tennis great Monica Seles. In her inspirational autobiography, *Getting a Grip*, Seles openly reveals the emotional turmoil around her eating disorder and the "courageous battle to find balance and harmony beyond tennis."[141]

Eating disorders go beyond emotional eating. Left untreated, physical symptoms of eating disorders can be serious. They can adversely affect athletic performance, not to mention normal growth and development in young women and men. The American Psychiatric Association uses standard diagnostic criteria for eating disorders, defined in their *Diagnostic and Statistical Manual of Mental Disorders (DSM)*.[142] The *DSM* defines the following eating disorders:

**Anorexia nervosa** is self-imposed starvation with an obsessive effort to lose weight to become thin. This disturbed body self-image can lead to severely low body weight, dehydration, and malnutrition.

**Bulimia** is recurring binge eating, the consumption of an extreme number of calories, followed by some method of purging, such as vomiting, laxative abuse, excessive exercise, or diuretic use.

**Bulimarexia** is anorexia nervosa with practice of bulimic behaviors.

The National Eating Disorders Association (NEDA) suspects the incidence of eating disorders is much higher in athletes, particularly females.[143] According to the ACSM, the National Collegiate Athletic Association (NCAA) shows that over 40 percent of their colleges and universities reported at least one case of anorexia or bulimia in their athletic programs. Approximately 90 percent of the reports were in women's sports.[144] Men can experience eating disorders too, but they do so less frequently than women. Tennis players cannot be excluded from this statistic. NEDA identifies risk factors for eating disorders in athletes.

---

The following risk factors could affect eating disorders in young tennis players (NEDA):

- an overvalued belief that lower body weight will improve performance
- sports that focus on the individual rather than the team

- psychosocial issues, including low self-esteem; parents who live through the success of their child; peer, family, and cultural pressures to be thin; family members who engage in chronic dieting or have an eating disorder; history of traumatic life experience, such as physical or sexual abuse
- coaches who focus primarily on success and performance rather than the athlete as a whole person
- training for a sport since childhood or being an elite athlete, such as a tennis player[145]

Signs and symptoms of eating disorders can appear as early as childhood, throughout teen and collegiate years, and continue through adulthood. Eating disorders can come as no surprise in the tennis circuit. The pressure of a driven athlete's quest for winning directly relies on his or her body weight and physical fitness level. Combined with additional risks (such as depression, anxiety, bipolar illness, low self-esteem, and distorted body image leading to an intense fear of gaining weight), an eating disorder could result.

Many athletes with eating disorders may erroneously believe that a thin physique and low body-fat percentage are the cornerstones to athletic performance. Just the opposite—physical symptoms of eating disorders not only impair sports performance but, more seriously, can stunt growth and development in children and teens. Withdrawing food and nutrients, in the case of anorexia nervosa, affects athletic performance by causing light-headedness; fatigue; loss of muscular strength, endurance, and coordination; and impaired focus and judgment. Starvation also affects growth and development, causing amenorrhea (disruption of menstrual cycle) and osteoporosis, leading to painful stress fractures. Stress fractures are microfractures of the bones that can progress to complete fractures.

The female athlete triad is a syndrome defined by the interrelated components of low energy availability, amenorrhea, and osteoporosis.[146] Energy availability is defined as caloric intake minus energy expenditure from exercise. When this balance causes net energy availability to be too low, disruptions can occur in menstrual function and bone health. The female athlete triad may or may not be related to disordered eating.

This syndrome can compromise nutritional status, physical performance, and immune function. At its extreme, the female athlete triad can lead to serious injuries, even mortality in young female athletes. Coaches, trainers, sports psychologists, and RDs working with physically active girls and young women should educate themselves to recognize and manage the female athlete triad.[147]

Eating disorders also bring a myriad of psychosocial concerns to the affected individual as well as to family, friends, and coaches. Like parents, coaches have a critically important role in identifying and looking for warning signs of eating disorders. The NEDA website (www.NationalEatingDisorders.org) is an excellent resource for coaches and parents. By all means, parents and coaches need to seek medical attention, psychological support, and nutritional care if an eating disorder is suspected in their child or teen tennis player.

## Weight Management Scenario #2: The Breakfast Skipper

You have heard that breakfast is the most important meal of the day. There are a number of reasons for this. As we sleep, we are fasting and utilizing glycogen stores in our liver to sustain blood sugar levels. When we awake, we should restore these glycogen reserves by eating or "breaking the fast" for adequate energy to start our active morning. This is especially important for the athlete who will draw on these glycogen stores during physical activity.

Many dieters think they are saving calories by skipping breakfast. I have worked with so many individuals who genuinely believe that skipping breakfast is doing more help than harm by saving them calories. True, the calories are not consumed, but the bigger impact of breakfast skipping is well documented. Studies show that breakfast skippers may actually consume more calories than their breakfast-eating counterparts by overeating during the day and having poorer quality diets.[148] Breakfast skippers tend to gain weight over time.[149]

Immediate impact of skipping breakfast includes morning irritability, lack of energy, and difficulty focusing. Drink a cup of coffee or two on an empty early morning stomach and add jitteriness, anxiety, and trips to the bathroom to the breakfast skipper's list of woes—not to mention the morning tennis game.

Breakfast is not only important for adults. Study after study show that eating breakfast improves academic performance in school-aged children.[150] Eating a breakfast meal with protein results in increased mental alertness and focus—essential for success in the classroom and on the tennis court.

It goes without saying that breakfast should serve up significant nutrition, actually up to one-third of the nutrients our bodies need. Carbohydrates provide energy and replenish glycogen stores for the steady, readily available fuel needed for optimal athletic performance. Protein and fat provide amino acids and fatty acids. Protein and fat also promote satiety or the feeling of fullness to stave off hunger pangs and satisfy appetite. Midmorning tennis cannot be successful when played with a grumbling stomach and hazy brain. Essential vitamins, minerals, fiber, and phytonutrients come from common breakfast foods like whole-grain cereal, yogurt, and fruit.

The realities of a busy, active day can cause hurried or even missed meals. One common reason people skip breakfast is lack of time. Tennis players are often on the go, attending school, practicing, training in the early morning hours, or going to work.

Despite hectic early morning schedules, breakfast can be made simple through quick-and-easy selections. Utilize these tips to make breakfast a priority. It should come as natural as taking a shower or brushing your teeth.

- **"Timing is everything."** Many folks are not hungry very early in the morning but may be ready to eat on their commute or arrival at school or the office. Many schools offer breakfast options. Between school periods, walk to class with a breakfast bar, yogurt parfait, or smoothie. At the office; during the work commute, in the car, bus, or subway; at the staff lounge; locker room or tennis court, eat a balanced breakfast to give you the energy needed to take on the day. No matter where you are or where you go, eat breakfast. Utilize the ideas below for on-the-go breakfast.
- **Pack it.** A simple, healthy breakfast consisting of yogurt and fruit can travel well to the tennis court, school, or work. Wash down with single-serve 100 percent fruit juice. Other simple, healthy, on-the-go breakfast ideas include the following:
  - oatmeal, dried fruit, and walnuts—instant oatmeal is easy to prepare and still provides whole-grain nutrition
  - breakfast protein bar and a banana, apple, or peach
  - bagel with light cream cheese, spinach leaves, and tomato
  - baggies or boxes of whole-grain cereal and milk. Milk can be kept in the office refrigerator or purchased at school; nonperishable individual serving-sized boxes of soy milk come in handy
  - yogurt and fresh berries with granola
  - peanut-butter-and-jam sandwich on whole-grain bread

- **Store it.** Keep healthy breakfast options in your tennis bag, office desk drawer, or locker. Bars are an on-the-go necessity—breakfast, granola, protein, and whole-grain cereal bars are good examples. Carry cans, boxes, or bottles of 100 percent juice, packets of nuts and raisins, trail mix, and whole fresh and dried fruit, which travel well whether in a briefcase, backpack, or tennis bag.

Another common reason people do not eat breakfast is because they feel full—as a result of overeating the night before to curb their hunger from skipped breakfast the morning before. It becomes a vicious cycle. Eating breakfast can break this cycle.

When meals are skipped, the body (and brain) may overcompensate by consuming more calories later in the day and evening. Although subject to expert debate, late-night eating can be especially deleterious to weight, because we consume a disproportionate number of calories at a time we are most sedentary. To make matters worse, these nighttime calories may be coming from junk foods that are low in nutrition and high in calories. There is little opportunity to burn these excess calories when we retire for sleep, only to wake up the next morning feeling full. To break this cycle, minimize late-night eating. Over several days, your body and brain will be ready to eat breakfast, breaking this cycle once and for all.

## Weight Management Scenario #3: The Chronic Dieter

The chronic dieter attempts to lose weight by focusing on diet alone and may or may not add exercise to his or her weight-loss regimen. Reducing calories, often through extremely low-calorie diets, causes pounds to shed. However, this weight frequently comes back as fast as it left, once unhealthy eating behaviors resume and sedentary lifestyle habits continue.

From the Paleo diet to raw foods to garcinia cambogia, there are hundreds, probably thousands, of diet plans hitting the fad-diet time line. Interestingly, the first fad diet goes back to the 1820s, when both the vinegar and water and the low-carbohydrate diet were in vogue. Yes. The low-carbohydrate diet dates to the early nineteenth century, weaving in and out of the fad-diet time line for almost two hundred years![151]

I have worked with many clients who have tried countless fad diets to quickly lose weight for a wedding, party, or high school reunion—even a tennis match—not understanding the physiological repercussions of sudden caloric restriction and weight loss on their bodies. Chronic dieters seek the next auspicious answer to permanent weight loss. For these individuals, dieting may be a temporary fix, addressing what we eat, but not why and how we eat the way we do.

Chronic dieting is detrimental to our bodies. In the absence of exercise or physical activity, low-calorie diets cause our metabolic rate (the rate at which we burn calories) to become sluggish. This is the exact opposite of what we want our metabolism to do, which is to more efficiently burn calories. The leaner our bodies, the more efficiently we can burn calories from food for energy. Exercise and strength training preserve and build muscle mass—no diet alone can do that. Diets that claim to build muscle or increase metabolism are not truthful, leading hopeful consumers to deception and disappointment.

Change perspective about food. Rather than focusing on excluding a wide range of foods or food groups from your diet, think inclusively by eating a wide variety of foods in moderation. Chronic dieters need to keep the age-old expression in mind: there is no such thing as a bad food, only bad eating habits.

If diets don't work, how do people lose weight and keep it off? The National Weight Control Registry (NWCR), established in 1994, is the largest study of long-term successful weight management. The NWCR tracks thousands of individuals who have lost weight and have been able to successfully keep it off. Their investigation supports the fact that the most successful participants kept weight off through long-term lifestyle changes, primarily good diet and high levels of physical activity. Registry members have lost an average of sixty-six pounds and have kept it off for over five years.[152]

Other facts about these successful NWCR members include the following:

- Ninety-eight percent modified their food intake in an effort to lose weight, with most reporting to maintain a lower-calorie, low-fat diet and doing high levels of activity.
- Ninety-four percent increased their physical activity.
- Ninety percent exercised, on average, about one hour per day.
- Seventy-eight percent ate breakfast every day.
- Sixty-two percent watched fewer than ten hours of television a week.[153]

(NWCR, www.nwcr.ws)

## WEIGHT MANAGEMENT SCENARIO #4: THE UNINFORMED OR MISINFORMED EATER

Since nutrition has become such a popular hotbed for dialogue, everyone seems to have an opinion about food and often erroneous opinions on nutrition. Some folks are simply misinformed, some folks are uninformed, and some just simply think they are nutrition know-it-alls. They have yet to acknowledge or accept that simple changes in their diet can make a tremendous difference in their weight and tennis play.

Some people have a difficult time managing weight because they do not know what to do or what to eat. Many will make the right move to seek professional guidance.

This can be described better by several cases in point. Megan, a friend of mine and an outstanding singles player, wanted to lose five pounds for an upcoming USTA tennis playoff match she and her 4.5 ladies team proudly earned during the regular season of play. Megan was to play singles, midday July, in Orlando, Florida. To intensify her need for physical conditioning and playoff pressure, she was to play on the blistery hot and fast hard court, a surface she was not used to playing on. She was used to playing on slower Har-Tru courts. When I asked Megan basic questions about her nutrition, I noted she used 2 percent milk, always had an evening sweet treat to satisfy her late-night sweet tooth (such as cookies or brownies) and, on occasion, skipped breakfast. The remainder of her eating pattern was sound.

I suggested a gradual switch to 1 percent, skim or fortified, low-fat soy milk; gave her suggestions of healthier food options to satisfy her evening sweet tooth and for being mindful about the cause of this evening cue; and insisted she always eat breakfast not only for nutrition but for high-energy tennis performance. Coupled with the additional exercise from her team's tennis practices, these simple changes led her to meet her realistic goal of losing five pounds (and keeping it off) before her big playoff match. This modest weight loss made big gains for her movement and confidence on the hard court.

Lane, another tennis friend of mine, was also trying to lose weight. In a casual conversation on the tennis court, Lane readily admitted he was a cola addict. He drank about twelve to fourteen cans of regular cola each day, equal to a whopping 1,800 calories and 108 teaspoons of table sugar (actually, high fructose corn syrup), not to mention caffeine, phosphoric acid, and artificial coloring. Before I could respond, he proclaimed he disliked diet cola, adamantly refusing to stomach it. Incidentally, Lane towers over six foot three and weighed 243 pounds.

I explained how much high fructose corn syrup, caffeine, and empty calories were in his daily dose of soda, along with the impact this had on his weight, blood sugar, and insulin levels, not to mention tennis performance. He paid heed by gradually reducing his daily cola intake. He is now down to a moderate one to two cans per day. Lane surely knew his soda drinking was detrimental to his health, but he needed someone else to reinforce the behavior change by not only discouraging soda intake but also encouraging healthy drink options for hydration—those he would like.

This simple change resulted in huge gains in his health. Lane lost over twenty pounds in a period of four months and has since kept the weight off for good. He met his goal weight target of 225 pounds on his birthday—the best gift he has ever received. Because he was getting an exorbitantly high number of calories from soda, the weight quickly came off. He substituted soda with water and diluted juice for hydration. He wisely coupled this major diet change with routine exercise at the gym. He became more fit, advanced to his next USTA level, and was club mixed doubles champ a few months later—great returns on investment for making this simple switch.

It can be easy for people to overlook simple changes in their diet for a number of reasons. Admittedly, some folks have a very difficult time changing or undoing bad eating habits and behaviors—they are, understandably, hard to let go. They may resort to other more appealing weight-loss options. Diets promising instant weight loss and perfect health are alluring. By resorting to unsound diet plans, they make weight management way more complicated than it has to be.

Whether you are a club or elite tennis player trying to manage your weight, seek advice from a professional. RDs and CSSDs can provide sound counseling advice, providing practical, realistic suggestions to help you lose weight and keep it off. They can come up with a mutually agreeable plan, individualized around your personal needs, such as work/training schedule, food preferences, food allergies, and exercise and fitness goals. They (and you) can explore reasons why you eat the way you do, affecting long-term behavioral changes for better weight and health outcomes. With proper guidance, successful weight management may be much simpler than many of us make it out to be.

# 7

# HYDRATION FOR OPTIMAL TENNIS PERFORMANCE

**Tennis is a perfect combination of violent action
taking place in an atmosphere of total tranquility.**
—Billie Jean King

Marcus, an excellent club tennis player, struggles to drink enough fluids, both on and off the court. Feeling sluggish right before a league playoff singles match, he thought he would fulfill his need for both fluids and a jolt of energy by guzzling down a twenty-four-ounce energy drink. "If these drinks work for X Games athletes, why not try it out for tennis?" he rationalized. Already feeling uneasy about his match, Marcus's anxiety level intensified after chugging down his energy drink. As he walked on the court, he felt his heart race and his breathing accelerate. Was it more than adrenaline racing through his body? Yes. It was the caffeine, sugars, and additives in his energy drink. Marcus downed his drink too quickly to give his body time to metabolize its potent ingredients. Unable to control his body's response, as if it were turning against him, Marcus made countless unforced errors throughout his once high-percentage tennis game. Anxious and on the edge, he found it difficult to concentrate and focus.

Marcus was also not drinking enough water between his games. He ended up losing his match, and has never forgotten that uncontrollable feeling on the court.

## THE SCIENCE OF SWEAT AND THIRST

Tennis hydration has come a long way from gulping pickle juice or water laced with a couple of salt tablets from a tennis ball can. Like nutrition, hydration is the other critical component of the sports nutritional science equation. Hydration during tennis is essential not only for peak performance but also for health and safety.

During exercise, muscles contract and generate heat. Core and skin temperatures increase. This heat is dissipated by perspiration or sweating. Sweating is the body's adaptive response to cool itself. The average adult has two to four million sweat glands. As sweat evaporates, our bodies cool. The combination of tennis played in a hot climate on a sweltering tennis court causes the body to sweat at an accelerated rate. Sweat losses on hot, humid days of tennis play can be substantial.

Besides containing water, sweat contains many other minerals. These include sodium, chloride, magnesium, calcium, and potassium. Sweat also contains ammonia, lactate, urea, zinc, iron, copper, calcium, chromium, nickel, and lead.

Sodium and chloride are the predominate minerals in sweat. They help maintain fluid balance, relax muscles, and help nerves transmit signals. Sodium and potassium are essential for electrical impulses to travel along nerves in order for muscles to contract—the ones engaged in prolonged tennis play. Our bodies need sodium and potassium in sufficient amounts for muscles to function.

When we lose more sodium and potassium in our sweat than

we can take in through food and fluids, muscle cramping can happen. Sodium is lost in sweat in a much greater quantity than potassium. Cramping is most frequently experienced in long, physically intense tennis matches played in hot weather. When the thermometer is high, so too are sweat rates, along with sodium and potassium losses.

Thirst is the body's physiological signal to drink fluids. As a result of fluid loss through sweat, the blood becomes more concentrated. This triggers the thirst mechanism, which causes the urge to drink. Drinking fluids brings the blood concentration back to normal levels. This proper fluid balance (fluids in equal fluids out) maintains blood volume. When blood volume is normal, blood is supplied to the skin for body temperature regulation. Since exercise produces heat, which must be eliminated from the body to maintain normal body temperatures, fluid intake is essential for cooling the body.

Because thirst cues lag behind the body's hydration needs, it is important to keep up with fluid replacement before thirst sets in. Hydrate before, during, and after a tennis match. Older tennis players (generally older than sixty) have an age-related blunting of thirst, making them more susceptible to dehydration.[154] This dulled thirst sensation can delay fluid intake even further. Combined with medications that affect fluid balance, elderly tennis players need to be vigilant about adequate hydration.

This age-related blunting of thirst recently struck a tennis friend of mine who had a near-miss case of heat exhaustion. Charlie, who is approaching seventy-one years old, was practicing singles with his opponent on a midmorning in July at our tennis club in Sarasota, Florida. As one would expect, July in southwest Florida is sizzling hot. This day also happened to be sunny and humid, with little cloud cover and a dearth of breeze or shade for reprieve. Consequently, the heat index was high.

Charlie thought he was drinking enough fluids to keep up with his copious sweat loss, but dizziness, nausea, and light-headedness quickly overcame him. Fortunately, he was playing with a cardiologist, who wisely advised him to get out of the heat, hydrate, and find air-conditioned refuge in the pro shop. With cooling towels on his head and neck, Charlie immediately felt better. Had he not done this, he could have collapsed from heat exhaustion.

## DEHYDRATION AND TENNIS

When dehydration happens, physiological strain on the body occurs. This strain can be serious. Body core temperature rises and heart rate increases. When dehydration hits the critical point of more than 2 percent of body weight lost, our brain loses cognitive/mental focus, particularly in hot environments.[155]

Heat exhaustion, heat cramps, and heat stroke are three types of heat-related illness. Dehydration increases the risk for these heat-related illnesses. Heat exhaustion is the result of the body overheating. Its symptoms are just as Charlie experienced, including heavy sweating, rapid pulse, fatigue, nausea, headache, dizziness, and faintness. Heat exhaustion is less severe than heat stroke but more severe than heat cramps.

Heat cramps are the mildest form of heat-related illness. However, they can be fatal to tennis performance. They are a symptom of heat exhaustion. The most accepted cause of heat cramps is dehydration, resulting in electrolyte loss, particularly sodium, chloride, and potassium. Another theory is that as muscles tire in the heat, they lose control of their own contractions, leading to the painful jerking movements many of us have experienced ourselves.[156]

Heat cramps are intermittent, involuntary spasms of large muscles that occur when athletes are physically active. The large muscles that most commonly cramp in tennis players are those in the legs and thighs. Cramping also plagues muscles in the arms and the core or abdomen. It is no wonder that heat cramps are a feared nemesis in the tennis world.

Heat cramps can usually be treated on the tennis court. If you suffer heat cramps, stop playing tennis and find a cool, shady place to rest. In more elite levels of play, you may have seen trainers or coaches gently stretch the affected player's muscles. This is also helpful in treating muscle cramps. As expected, fluids and electrolytes need to be replaced by drinking water, sports drinks, and electrolyte solutions. In more extreme cases, intravenous (IV) fluid solutions need to be given. Seek medical care if heat cramps cannot be controlled and other symptoms like nausea, vomiting, fatigue, and weakness develop. Tennis players who have experienced heat cramps are at risk for having them again.

If left to progress, the most severe heat-related illness, heat stroke, can occur. Heat stroke is a medical emergency that can be fatal at its extreme. The body is no longer able to cool itself. Bodily temperature could reach 106 degrees, leading to slurred speech, confusion, and imminent coma. Heat stroke requires immediate medical attention.

Dehydration also increases the risk of rhabdomyolysis. Rhabdomyolysis is a syndrome causing breakdown and release of muscle contents into the bloodstream during physical overexertion. Rhabdomyolysis can cause the kidneys to work so hard to eliminate the waste products of muscle breakdown they go in to acute kidney failure. Although rhabdomyolysis is rare in the tennis world, know that this life-threatening syndrome can be prevented with proper hydration.

Elderly amateur athletes are not alone. Even young, highly trained professional athletes have succumbed to heat cramping and heat exhaustion. The world has watched the most decorated professional athletes wither from heat cramps. National Basketball Association (NBA) Cleveland Cavaliers superstar and former Miami Heat champion LeBron James had a very public episode of heat cramping during the 2014 NBA playoff games against the San Antonio Spurs. Playing hard in a warm arena during an air conditioner malfunction, coupled with a lack of fluids, caused the downfall of one of basketball's all-time top players.

Peng Shuai and Steve Johnson dodged their hopes for a shot at the 2014 US Open title due to heat cramps and heat exhaustion. Shuai was in the women's semifinal match against Caroline Wozniacki when heat cramps suddenly overcame her. Heat exhaustion caused Shuai to retire from her most successful US Open.

Facets of tennis create the perfect storm for inducing heat-related illness. Not only is tennis mostly played outdoors in hot climates, the duration of match play is unpredictable. A two-set match can last anywhere from an effortless one hour to a tumultuous three hours. Unlike the breaks between boxing rounds or on the football field sidelines, there are no coaches or trainers who handily provide fluids to tennis players. We are on our own.

In addition, the type of tennis played influences fluid need, consequently the potential for heat-related illness. Exercise duration and intensity have the greatest impact on fluid replacement needs.[157] Doubles tennis will not require as much fluid replacement as the same duration of singles tennis, since exercise intensity is much greater in singles than in doubles tennis.

Even style of tennis play influences fluid (and nutrient) needs on and off the court. As an example, tennis players who engage in the baseline rally style of play will expend more energy than players who quickly come to net to "put the ball away" and end the point. Some players like to shorten points; some like to stretch them out. A three-hour singles match chasing down countless balls requires more fluids than a ninety-minute match characterized by shorter points. Recognize your tennis style and scout your opponent's— then match your hydration needs accordingly.

Environment has a tremendous impact on the body's temperature regulation. Hands down, hot, humid weather combined with intense tennis will significantly augment fluid needs in both doubles and singles play. This is because our bodies need to dissipate heat produced from both exercise and hot ambient temperature. Ensure proper hydration in cooler weather too. Sweating still occurs under layers of clothing. Because sweat is quickly absorbed with winter wear, while evaporating more quickly on exposed areas, this may mask our need to hydrate. Always hydrate during tennis, in both hot and cooler climates.

## FLUID REQUIREMENTS FOR TENNIS

Have you been told to drink eight cups of water each day, twelve cups, or maybe even a gallon? If so, be discriminating about these "one size fits all" recommendations, especially if you are a competitive tennis player. Without knowing the duration of a tennis match, coupled with the many determinants of fluid requirements, fluid needs can be substantially more (or fewer) than eight cups or twelve cups or a gallon per day—tennis players need to be prepared for that.

Like nutrient needs, fluid needs must be individualized. A number of factors influence fluid needs:

1. **Body Weight.** The more an individual weighs, generally, the more calories and fluid needed. A larger person has more body surface area, demanding greater fluid intake.
2. **Gender.** Women tend to sweat less than men because they have lower body weight and metabolism.[158] Metabolism is the rate at which calories are burned.
3. **Climate.** The hotter or more humid the climate, the more an individual will perspire. Fluid and electrolytes lost in sweat in hot climate can be significant. Don't be deceived—heated indoor air in the wintertime can also cause skin to lose significant moisture. Since tennis is most often played outdoors in a sunny, warm climate, fluid losses can be very high.

4. **Heat Acclimatization.** You probably have experienced moving to a new environment with its accompanying climate. Adjusting to a new climate—particularly a hotter, more humid one—takes the body time to become heat acclimatized. Heat acclimatization enhances an individual's ability to adapt to a new environment. In hotter climates, acclimatization helps athletes achieve higher and more sustained sweat rates when needed. Tennis players who are heat acclimatized may sweat more (or less) than their nonacclimatized counterparts and have a better "read" of their fluid needs.

5. **Altitude.** Altitudes greater than 8,200 feet may trigger increased urination and more rapid breathing, which will cause you to lose more fluids. This is because at higher altitudes, lower air pressure makes it more difficult for oxygen to enter our systems. We respond by breathing more rapidly to get more oxygen in our bodies. When we are unable to get enough oxygen even to do simple physical tasks, the result is shortness of breath, dizziness, nausea, and fatigue.

Physical activity becomes difficult. Many tennis players will feel the difference when they play in geographic regions of higher altitudes (e.g., one to two miles above sea level). Acclimatization to higher altitude environments will help the body adapt more efficiently, whether it is social play or elite, competitive play. Be prepared to adjust your nutrient and fluid intake when playing in high altitudes.

6. **Physical Activity/Exercise.** Exercise and physical activity are the single greatest determinants of fluid losses and fluid replacement needs. How much fluid you need depends on how much you sweat during exercise as well as the intensity, duration, and type of exercise.

7. **Sweat Rate.** Different individuals have different sweat rates that influence fluid loss and the fluid required to make up the deficit. This is apparent on and off the court. Some individuals you know may sweat profusely during activity or stress, while others are cool as a cucumber. Sweat rates can typically range from one to four pounds per hour, the equivalent of 480–2,000 milliliters of fluid lost in sweat.[159] This is a tremendous range, making it challenging to prescribe a "one size fits all" recommendation for fluid intake.

8. **Illness or Health Problems.** Fever, vomiting, and diarrhea cause your body to lose fluids. In more severe cases, intravenous solutions may be necessary to replace fluid and electrolytes. Any disease or illness, such as a urinary tract infection, that causes you to lose fluid would necessitate more fluid replacement.

The most accurate way to determine fluid replacement needs due to sweat loss from tennis is to weigh yourself before a training session and then afterward. The difference in weight will be the amount of sweat lost and, consequently, the fluid required to replace this loss. Over a 1 percent loss in body weight indicates dehydration. For example, if you weigh 180 pounds prior to a tennis match or practice and weigh 178 pounds afterward, you would be experiencing dehydration, evidenced by a greater than 1 percent weight loss. Refer to the table below to assess your fluid status based on pre- and postexercise weight.[160]

Be sure to weigh yourself exactly the same way before and after exercise. One pound of sweat equates to approximately 480 milliliters of fluid loss. For competitive players, engage the assistance of a certified athletic trainer to more closely measure sweat rate and the fluids required to replace sweat loss. Good hydration can mean the difference between a match win or loss. Most importantly, good hydration is important for overall health.

**Table 7.1: Percent Body Weight Change and Hydration Status (Source: Simpson & Howard, ACSM)**

| Hydration Status | Percent Body Weight Change |
|---|---|
| Well Hydrated | -1 to +1 percent |
| Minimal Dehydration | -1 to -3 percent |
| Significant Dehydration | -3 to -5 percent |
| Serious Dehydration | > -5 percent |

The next best indicator of whether or not fluid replacement needs have been met is to check urine color, volume, and odor. If your urine is a concentrated dark yellow or amber color, scant in volume, and/or has a strong odor, your fluid intake has fallen way short of replacement needs. Dark amber-colored urine indicates dehydration. Urine color should be light straw colored to nearly clear, indicating that fluid needs have been met through proper hydration. Keep in mind that certain medications, vitamins, and supplements may cause a darkening or urine color change. Utilize urine color charts to help you evaluate your hydration status. These may be conveniently posted in your tennis club's restroom.

## ABOUT FLUIDS: HOW MUCH DO I NEED?

**1. Baseline Fluid Needs.** Total fluid needs include baseline needs plus added fluid, determined by the many factors listed above. Baseline fluid needs meet the body's basic requirements for metabolism, digestion, circulation, and excretion. Once these baseline fluid needs are calculated, additional fluid must be added for exercise and the other influences, including sweat rate.

Baseline fluid needs can be calculated a number of ways. There are acceptable formulas to calculate baseline fluid needs in adults. One common rule of thumb is to calculate one milliliter of fluid per every calorie consumed.

Example: If you consume two thousand calories per day, your

baseline fluid need would be two thousand milliliters, to which you add extra fluids to replace sweat loss from exercise.

**2. Additional Fluid Needs for Exercise.** Recognizing that most individuals lose in the range of 480–2,000 milliliters of sweat per hour during exercise and considering the many other determinants of fluid need (gender, climate, exercise intensity and duration, etc.), individual fluid requirements are highly variable between players. In extremely hot weather, tennis players can lose up to five thousand milliliters of sweat per hour, the equivalent to five liters of fluid, sodium, magnesium, potassium, and other important minerals and electrolytes. Providing generic recommendations for fluids—those eight glasses of water a day—is ineffectual. On hot days of tennis play, drinking an additional two liters or more of water and/or sports drink during your match can be expected.

Drinking 120–240 milliliters of water for every fifteen minutes of strenuous exercise, like singles tennis in hot climate, is a general recommendation to safeguard against under hydration. If you sweat profusely, your fluid needs can be double the amount, or 240–480 milliliters, of water for every fifteen minutes of strenuous exercise.[161]

Odd-game tennis breaks lend themselves nicely to support adequate hydration. At every tennis break between odd games, always hydrate—no exceptions. Ranchordas suggests competitive tennis players consume two hundred milliliters of fluid containing electrolytes in every changeover in mild to moderate temperatures of 27° C, or 80.6° F. In temperatures greater than 27° C, tennis players should aim for less than or equal to four hundred milliliters.[162] Keep in mind the long list of determinants of fluid needs outlined above. Your fluid needs will be more or less, considering these influences.

Gauge your fluid intake by taking a bathroom break between sets. Once again, if your urine is scant, dark, and concentrated, you need to drink more fluids. If your urine is nearly clear with a tinge of color and has volume, you are hydrating enough.

# FLUIDS: WHAT TO DRINK, WHEN, AND WHY

**Water.** Water is king of fluids, reigning as the original sports drink. Fifty percent of the body is composed of water. Water transports nutrients, eliminates waste products, regulates body temperature (through sweating), and maintains blood pressure and circulation. Water is the best beverage to drink during exercise to replace water losses from sweat. Water should be sufficient to replace fluids in the first sixty minutes of strenuous tennis activity, such as continual drilling and singles match play.

Water can be bland tasting for tennis players, particularly teens and children. Adults may feel the same way. As a consequence, we may bypass water as the fluid of choice over more appealing, colorful, sugar-sweetened beverages and sports drinks. In addition, we may stop drinking water before we are fully hydrated. Make a concerted effort to ensure your fluid needs are met by water.

To enhance water's appeal, spice it up with flavor. Many companies now make flavor drops to add a hint of taste to water. Adding a squeeze of fresh lemon, orange, or lime juice provides citrusy refreshment. Infusing water with berries, citrus slices, or cucumber adds pizzazz. Sprigs of mint or other fresh herbs can also add enough appeal to encourage drinking this healthiest beverage for hydration and sports performance.

Engineered sport powders and drops can provide electrolytes, carbohydrates, vitamins, minerals, and other supplements. These are useful when exercise exceeds an hour, when our bodies necessitate repletion of carbohydrates and electrolytes. Follow the package directions when mixing these ergogenic aids to water.

Designer bottled waters that have undergone special processes from vapor distillation, osmosis, alkalinization, and electrolyte infusion have become very popular. Again, the main function of bottled water is hydration. If these specialized waters cause you to drink more fluids before, during, and after a tennis match to stay hydrated, then go for them.

*Bottled or Tap?* Over half of Americans drink bottled water—54 percent to be exact, per the National Resources Defense Council.[163] In 2014 sales of bottled water tipped close to $13 billion and continue to grow.[164] Bottled water is in high demand, becoming the expected mode of delivery for our drinking water.

Much of the appeal of bottled water is the perception that it supplies a safer, higher-quality source of water compared to tap water. The Environmental Protection Agency (EPA) regulates the purity and sanitation of tap water, while the Food and Drug Administration (FDA) regulates bottled water. The EPA regulates the levels of ninety different contaminants, including germs, heavy metals, lead, and industrial chemicals, which can vary from region to region. Tap water is safe to drink, although it can taste different from bottled water.

Bottled water and tap water can come from the same exact source: lakes, springs, and water plants. Much of the bottled water we drink is tap water that has been filtered and treated with extra steps to taste better. If the taste of bottled water encourages you to hydrate more, by all means choose bottled water over tap water. If filtered tap water is palatable, you can reap the benefits of hydration with this inexpensive water source, carried to the courts in your reusable water jug.

Incidentally, the demand for bottled water has made a significant environmental impact. Bottled water has resulted in an additional fifty billion plastic bottles per year, of which only a fraction—less than 20 percent—are recycled. The remaining 80 percent, or forty billion bottles, end up in landfills or as pollution in our land, oceans, lakes, and streams.[165] If this is a concern of yours, use your reusable jug with your own water filled just the way you like it.

**Sports Drinks.** For exercise lasting anywhere between sixty minutes or longer (such as a two-hour singles tennis match), sports drinks containing fluid, carbohydrates, and electrolytes are beneficial.[166] At this point of intense exercise duration, both fluids and electrolytes lost in sweat should be replaced through sports drinks for optimal athletic performance. Hot tennis climate increases sweat and electrolyte loss during exercise—common weather for tennis play—making sports drinks very useful. Sports drinks restore the carbohydrates, or fuel, that have been used up in intense physical exercise.

The carbohydrates in sports drinks provide quick energy to muscles and the brain. According to the American College of Sports Medicine, the greatest rates of carbohydrate delivery to muscles can be achieved with a mixture of sugars: glucose, sucrose, fructose, and maltodextrin.[167] Evidence suggests that multiple types of carbohydrates in sports food and fluids get transported through different mechanisms, making the energy more available for use by working muscles.[168] These carbs can be used as an immediate fuel source for muscles and brain. Any carbohydrate not used for quick fuel can be stored, replacing the glycogen in muscles and liver already used up during exercise.

Many sports drinks on the market provide carbohydrates in the form of sucrose, glucose, and dextrose. These sports drinks deliver carbohydrates in the proper concentration of water without impeding the absorption of fluid. With the proper ratio of water to carbohydrates, water can be absorbed in a sports drink at the same rate as plain water.

Be wary of sports drinks with too high of a sugar content. A higher sugar concentration in a sports drink or any sugar-sweetened beverage can delay fluid or water absorption. For each molecule of sugar, it takes a molecule of water to digest it—this water is needed for hydration and should not be diverted to digest a sugary drink. Look for a sports drink providing no more than 6 percent carbohydrate concentration. This is equivalent to fourteen to sixteen grams per eight-ounce serving of sports drink. The following example helps calculate this ratio:

**Example 1: Sports Drink**—too high in carbohydrate concentration

8 oz. (= 240 ml or 240 g, one milliliter is approximately one gram)
Contains: 22 g carbohydrate per 8 oz. serving
22 gms ÷ 240 gms = 9 percent carbohydrate concentration
**Example 2: Sports Drink**—proper carbohydrate concentration
8 oz. (= 240 ml or 240 g)
Contains: 14 g carbohydrate per 8 oz. serving
14 gms ÷ 240 gms = 5.8 percent carbohydrate concentration, rounds up to 6 percent

During exercise lasting greater than sixty minutes, carbohydrate should be consumed at a rate of thirty to sixty grams per hour in a 6–8 percent carbohydrate solution every ten to fifteen minutes, equivalent to eight to sixteen ounces of sports drink.[169] In singles tennis played in a hot climate, hydrating with a sports drink and water at every changeover should be reflexive. Electrolytes (such as sodium, chloride, and potassium) in sports drinks replace those lost in sweat. Carbohydrates in the form of glucose, fructose, and maltodextrin continually fuel muscles.

Finding a sports drink that tastes good is a fairly easy task. Their bright-neon colors and appealing flavors have overtaken shelves in the beverage sections of stores. Especially attractive to children and teens, sports drinks may be chosen over water. As a reminder, for normal hydration need, in the absence of prolonged exercise (greater than sixty minutes) in hot climates, water remains the beverage of choice for hydration.

Sports drinks should be used for what they were designed to do—enhance sports performance during intense exercise. Since we get enough sodium in our diet—too much—drinking sports drinks at the school lunch or dinner table, shopping mall, or movie theater and on every occasion except during athletics only provides unneeded sodium. For adults and children watching their weight, the excess, unnecessary simple sugars and calories in sports drinks add empty calories with minimal nutrition.

Sugar-free sports drinks are low calorie because they use

nonnutritive sugar substitutes in place of simple sugars or carbohydrates. However, by eliminating these carbohydrates necessary for athletic performance, sugar-free sports drinks become expensive salt water with sugar substitute and electrolytes. This defeats the primary purpose of sports drinks in fueling our muscles with carbohydrates, before, during and after exercise.

**Energy Drinks.** Energy drinks have attracted tennis players among athletes all over the globe. Athletes appreciate the "kick" energy drinks provide toward enhancing alertness, vigilance, concentration, and reaction speed. Reviewing the information on the most popular energy drinks on the US market, most all contain filtered water, sugar, caffeine, B vitamins, and such additives as taurine, guarana, green tea extract, and yerba mate. B vitamins are needed for energy production during exercise. Taurine is an amino acid found in meat, fish, and poultry, proposed—though not proven—to improve athletic performance. Yerba mate, guarana, and green tea extract all contain caffeine. Green tea extract and yerba mate contain antioxidants.

Third-party studies have demonstrated the effectiveness of energy drinks on sports performance. Studies on one of the most popular energy drinks consumed worldwide and endorsed by a number of professional athletes and celebrities show their brand can improve concentration, focus, and reaction speed in specific sports like cycling.[170]

However, is it the energy drink or its components, carbohydrates and caffeine that result in its ergogenic benefit? The International Society of Sports Nutrition's (ISSN) position stand on energy drinks is based on a critical analysis of the safety and usefulness of these popular beverages. The ISSN's conclusions on energy drinks include the following:

- The primary ergogenic nutrients in most energy drinks are carbohydrate (sugars) and caffeine.

- The potential benefit of other additives in energy drinks remains to be determined.

- Consuming an energy drink ten to sixty minutes before exercise can improve mental focus, alertness, anaerobic performance, and/or endurance performance.

- Children and teens should consider energy drinks with parental approval and after reviewing the caffeine, sugar, and nutrient content contained in their energy drink.

- Consuming more than one serving per day of an energy drink can result in harmful side effects, including anxiety, sleeplessness, and high blood sugar.[171]

If you feel energy drinks work for your tennis game, choose them with the above considerations in mind. They should be consumed over a period of time (not guzzled) about ten to sixty minutes before a tennis match to most effectively utilize their components.

Energy drinks are not the same as sports drinks—even though they can easily be mistaken for such. Energy drinks are not designed to hydrate. Energy drinks energize, while sports drinks replenish water, carbohydrates, electrolytes, and minerals. Water or sports drinks should still be consumed with (or without) energy drinks before and during exercise.

In the scenario described at the beginning of the chapter, Marcus used a twenty-four-ounce energy drink for hydration prior to his tennis match, thinking this would give him a tennis performance edge; this was a serious mistake. To compound his hydration woes, he was not well hydrated to begin with. He guzzled this large can of energy drink over a couple of minutes, not giving his body enough time to break down, absorb, and use the carbohydrates, caffeine, vitamins, and additives. He did not hydrate enough with water before and during his match. Already feeling some anxiety and nerves about his big match, the caffeine in his energy drink made him feel even more anxious, with heart racing from epinephrine gone out of control, wreaking havoc on his mental and physical performance. To this day, Marcus will never forget his horrible hydration experiment. He has since changed his hydration practices before and during his tennis matches.

If used and timed properly, consuming an energy drink before tennis, along with water or sports drink for hydration, could enhance tennis performance. If you want to try an energy drink before (or during) tennis, always experiment during a practice session. Then you know what to expect, which will give you confidence and reassurance during a real match.

**Caffeine-Containing Beverages.** Caffeine is one of the most widely used legal stimulants in the world and the most widely used dietary ergogenic in the sports world.[172] Caffeine is found in coffee, tea, energy drinks, chocolate, cocoa, cola, and over-the-counter medications. Caffeine is quickly absorbed and shows up in our bodies thirty to sixty minutes after ingestion.

Studies on caffeine show that small amounts, equivalent to one eight-ounce cup of brewed coffee, or one hundred milligrams of caffeine, prior to exercise can improve stamina and alertness in endurance sports, such as marathon running and cycling.[173] Caffeine has also been shown to be highly effective for time-trial performance.[174]

As with endurance exercise, caffeine has also been demonstrated to improve performance during short-term intense exercise lasting approximately five minutes. Studies have shown caffeine to improve sports involving intermittent activity, including soccer and rugby.[175]

Caffeine increases the release of adrenaline in the blood. Adrenaline is a hormone that stimulates many bodily functions, including mental alertness. As a result, caffeine should enhance focus and reaction speed.

If you want to utilize caffeine for its ergogenic effect, experiment during a practice match. Sports scientists suggest three to nine milligrams per kilogram of body weight of caffeine taken thirty to ninety minutes prior to exercise studied in well-trained, elite endurance athletes in the running and cycling world.[176,177] This suggestion would not apply to club or recreational tennis players.

As an example, if you weigh 150 pounds, or 68.2 kilograms, and consume three milligrams of caffeine per kilogram of body weight, the amount would equal 205 milligrams of caffeine, which is equivalent to two eight-ounce cups of brewed coffee. Remember, there is no caffeine recommendation specific to tennis play. Tennis engages anaerobic bursts of energy (e.g., in serving, rushing in for a drop shot, or chasing down a lob). Since there is evidence suggesting that caffeine improves sprint performance in short-term anaerobic activity in other stop-and-go sports, caffeine may provide ergogenic benefit on the tennis court.

Be reminded, too much caffeine can cause anxiety and jitters—exactly what you don't need on match day. Popular caffeine-containing drinks from the coffee bar can also be very high in calories, refined sugar, and fat. Table 7.2 outlines caffeine content of various beverages from the Center for Science in the Public Interest (CSPI).[178] CSPI also identifies various foods and drugs containing caffeine on their helpful website: www.cspinet. org/new/cafchart.

**Table 7.2: The Caffeine Content of Various Beverages (Source: CSPI, Caffeine Content of Food and Drugs)**

|  | Amount (ounces) | Caffeine Content (mg) |
|---|---|---|
| Coffee, brewed | 8 | 108 |
| Coffee, instant | 8 | 57 |
| Dunkin' Donuts coffee | 14 (medium) | 178 |
| Panera coffee | 16.8 | 189 |
| McDonald's coffee | 12 (small) | 109 |

|  | Amount (ounces) | Caffeine Content (mg) |
|---|---|---|
| Starbucks coffee | 12 (tall) | 260 |
| Starbucks coffee | 16 (grande) | 330 |
| Starbucks coffee | 20 (venti) | 415 |
| Starbucks mocha frappuccino | 24 (venti) | 140 |
| K-cup coffee | 8 | 120 |
| Decaf coffee, brewed | 8 | 6 |
| Hot tea, brewed | 8 | 30–80 |
| Green tea, brewed | 8 | 35–60 |
| Iced tea, brewed | 8 | 47 |
| Espresso | 1.5 | 77 |
| Classic Coke | 12 | 34 |
| Diet Coke | 12 | 45 |
| Pepsi | 12 | 38 |
| Diet Pepsi | 12 | 36 |
| Mountain Dew | 12 | 54 |
| Red Bull | 8.46 | 80 |
| Monster energy drink | 16 | 160 |
| Rockstar energy drink | 16 | 160 |
| 5-Hour energy drink | 2 | 138 |
| Chocolate milk | 8 | 5 |

*Information used by permission through CSPI, Copyright Clearance Center, January, 2015*

Because of caffeine's proven ergogenic effect, the World Anti-Doping Association (WADA) has listed it as a controlled substance. Professional athletes are permitted to use caffeine, but with restrictions. WADA prohibits caffeine when it reaches twelve micrograms or more in a urine sample. The NCAA considers caffeine a prohibited substance in collegiate athletes when it reaches fifteen micrograms or more in urine samples.[179]

**Coconut Water.** Everyone seems to be "going coconuts" for coconuts. From coconut milk to coconut oil, coconuts are in the nutritional spotlight. Coconut water is the clear liquid in the center of young, green coconuts. Dubbed the "natural sports drink," coconut water contains carbohydrates, electrolytes, and antioxidants. Coconut water is much higher in potassium and lower in sodium than most sports drinks. Table 7.3 provides a side-by-side comparison of eight ounces of coconut water and sports drink.

**Table 7.3: Comparison of Coconut Water and Sports Drink**

| Nutrient | Coconut Water, 8 oz. | Sports Drink, 8 oz. |
|---|---|---|
| Calories | 40 | 50 |
| Carbohydrate (g) | 10 | 14 |
| Sodium (mg) | 45–60 | 110 |
| Potassium (mg) | 480 | 30 |
| Magnesium (mg) | 57 | 0 |
| Calcium (mg) | 55 | 0 |

Although coconut water is deemed "nature's sports drink," its profile is not exactly what athletes need in prolonged, intense exercise lasting over sixty minutes. Coconut water does not provide enough sodium, which is lost in large amounts in sweat in a hot climate. In prolonged exercise, coconut water does not provide enough carbohydrates compared to the equivalent amount of sports drink. Sports drinks are higher in carbohydrates and sodium and much lower in potassium than coconut water.[180]

Few studies have examined coconut water in sports performance, including tennis. In one 2012 study in the *Journal of the International Society of Sports Nutrition*, Kalman and his team compared bottled water, sports drink, coconut water, and coconut water from concentrate on measures of rehydration and physical performance after exercise. On four separate occasions, the men were given one of the four drinks after a sixty-minute bout of dehydrating treadmill exercise. They found no differences in rehydration and physical performance of exercise-trained men when they drank coconut water or sports drink. However, they found that the men experienced greater bloating and stomach upset with the coconut water and coconut water from concentrate drinks.[181] This study looked at rehydration and physical performance after exercise on subsequent bouts of exercise over different days. It did not evaluate exercise performance when these drinks were provided during exercise. More research needs to be done on the efficacy of coconut water, including for tennis players.

Many athletes supplement coconut water with the appropriate amount of salt to bump up the sodium and chloride content. Tennis players can also supplement their coconut water with additional carbohydrates from crackers or pretzels during their match. Many like the taste of coconut water better than other beverages, including sports drinks and water. If this is the case, coconut water supplemented with salt or a salty, carbohydrate-containing snack, like pretzels, meets the criteria in replacing fluid, carbohydrates, and sodium during prolonged, intense exercise.

American tennis professional John Isner is one of these athletes who stands by coconut water as his beverage of choice before, during and after play. John Isner credited coconut water for keeping him going during his epic eleven-hour Wimbledon match against Nicolas Mahut in 2010. In a June 25, 2013, *Huffington Post* article writer Terri Coles stated Isner drank coconut water prior to and during his matches to keep him from cramping. Isner confirmed that coconut water kept him from cramping during his historic match against Mahut.

Unlike caffeine-containing beverages and energy drinks,

coconut water does rehydrate. Coconut water is an outstanding beverage choice over sugary, caffeinated beverages for both athletes and nonathletes. For recreational exercise, coconut water is a good option for hydration and refreshment. For many, it tastes great. Many also like the fact that pure coconut water is unadulterated with additives. Coconut water is good source of potassium and can fill in the gap when potassium from fresh fruits and vegetables is lacking. Eight ounces of coconut water has more potassium than a large banana.

When used as a sports drink for prolonged, strenuous tennis, (lasting more than sixty minutes), coupled with extra sodium and carbohydrates from food, coconut water becomes the natural sports drink. If you pack a large bottle of coconut water in your tennis bag, be sure to use it to wash down snacks containing extra carbohydrates and sodium, like pretzels, saltine crackers, or salty cereal mix. Like with any new ergogenic beverage, try it out at a practice session, not during a momentous match.

**Nutrient-Enhanced Waters** may contain small amounts of carbohydrates, electrolytes, vitamins, minerals, and additives. They are commonly fortified, donning various vitamin profiles, including B vitamins for energy and vitamins C and E for immune function. Many contain additives, such as ginseng, gingko biloba, guarana, taurine, green tea flavoring, and carnitine, to name a few.

Too little research has been done to determine whether their supplementation has any beneficial effect on exercise and health. In the case of tennis performance, the answer is likely "No." Nutrient-enhanced water may contain hidden caffeine from guarana and green tea extract. Caffeine acts as a diuretic, making you lose fluid. Look for this ingredient on the label to determine whether you want to keep caffeine in or out of your body.

What these waters do provide is fluids and nutrition, making them a reasonable beverage option off the court, but their key components are not in the proper concentrations compared to the fluid, carbohydrates, and electrolytes in sports drinks. Stick to water and sports drinks during tennis. During recreational activity, nutrient-enhanced waters are a better choice over sugar-sweetened beverages, like soda.

**Juice.** Although fruit juice has carbohydrates, vitamins, minerals, phytonutrients, and electrolytes, it is not a good choice for sports hydration. The high natural or added sugars in juice reduce the rate of water absorption in the digestive tract. As a result, the body does not get hydrated fast enough. Fruit juice also contains a high number of calories in a small portion. Eight ounces of fruit juice can have a bulging 130 calories compared to eight ounces of coconut water, which has 45 calories, and reliable water with 0 calories.

You can still get the nutritional benefit of juice when diluted with water. Diluting juice also reduces its high calorie content. Use juice as an excellent flavor enhancer to encourage water intake. Add a splash of your favorite juice to a container of water to stay hydrated while getting some carbohydrates, flavor, and additional nutrition at the same time. Remember that this solution should not be mistaken as a sports drink substitute, which has a different composition.

**Carbonated soft drinks** are not a good option for hydration or good nutrition but may have ergogenic benefit on the tennis court. First, the cons of soda. Most brands of regular soda contain simple sugars in the form of high fructose corn syrup (HFCS). Virtually all the calories in regular soda come from sugars. One twelve-ounce can of regular cola contains the equivalent of nine teaspoons of sugar. A twenty-ounce bottle of regular cola contains the equivalent of fifteen teaspoons of sugar. A supersized sixty-four-ounce soda at the local convenience store contains a whopping forty-four teaspoons of sugar!

In 2013, Statista, a statistics portal, revealed Americans drank about forty-two gallons of soft drinks per capita.[182] They also report that the United States held 21.6 percent of the world's market share for soda, consuming over one-fifth of all the carbonated beverages produced worldwide that year. Although this amount is staggering, US soda consumption is actually down from years past.

Soda is the largest source of sugar in the diets of children and teens. Because children, teens, and young adult tennis players are especially drawn to soda, they need to realize the tremendous amount of added sugar they are drinking from empty liquid calories and the nutritious fluids they displace when they drink soda: water, milk, 100 percent fruit juice—to name a few.

## HIGH FRUCTOSE CORN SYRUP: IS IT BETTER OR WORSE THAN SUCROSE?

Many food and beverage manufacturers have replaced sucrose or table sugar with high fructose corn syrup (HFCS) in their sugary beverages like soda, teas, energy drinks, and fruit beverages. HFCS is a calorie-providing sweetener made from glucose syrup derived from corn. HFCS entered the American food supply in the 1970s.

Not to be confused with the naturally occurring fructose in fruits, vegetables, and honey, HFCS is a sugar added to foods and beverages. Other added sugars include white sugar, corn syrup, malt syrup, sorbitol, anhydrous dextrose, and molasses. The list of added sugars to our food goes on. Many foods and beverages with large amounts of added sugars are usually high in calories and low in nutrition, with sugary beverages being on top of that list. In contrast, foods with naturally occurring fructose, like fruits and vegetables, have high nutritional value. Milk, containing lactose, or milk sugar, also provides nutrition. Despite its critics giving it a tarnished reputation, milk is a very healthy beverage—far better than sugary beverages for its natural sugar, protein, vitamin, mineral, and electrolyte content.

HFCS is appealing to food manufacturers for a number of reasons. It is sweeter than sucrose or sugar—in fact, six times as sweet. It retains a longer shelf life in foods and beverages, and it is less expensive than other sweeteners. Since the US government subsidizes corn production while setting high tariffs on the importation of sugar, the American corn supply is plentiful. Consequently, HFCS is a cheaper sweetener for food manufacturers to add to sugar-sweetened beverages than sugar or sucrose derived from the sugarcane plant or sugar beets.[183]

HFCS starts out as cornstarch. Chemical processing breaks down cornstarch into its simpler sugars, glucose and fructose. On the surface, HFCS and table sugar (sucrose) look identical. Both consist of the same two simple sugars, fructose and glucose. They both have the exact same calories. However, the fructose and glucose in table sugar are chemically bonded. The body must digest sucrose to cleave this bond, break it down, and absorb fructose and glucose. In contrast, the fructose and glucose in HFCS is blended together, no bond, which means it does not need to be digested before it enters the bloodstream.[184]

Some experts scrutinize HFCS for its negative impact on weight and overall health. They propose the difference in the way the body metabolizes HFCS promotes obesity, insulin resistance, high triglyceride levels, and diabetes in a more pronounced way than table sugar, even though both sweeteners have the same calories per serving.[185] Controversy exists, because experts have yet to corroborate on this theory; they are fervently investigating it. The American Medical Association (AMA) and the Academy of Nutrition and Dietetics (AND) position statements reflect that HFCS has the same effect on weight as table sugar, with the qualification that more research is needed to study the health impact of HFCS.[186]

Ask professional health advocacy organizations and leading experts in nutrition, epidemiology, and public health, and their stance on HFCS is much more suspect. Their concern is that our bodies do indeed react differently to HFCS than to other types of sweeteners.[187]

Although experts debate the health impact of table sugar versus HFCS, they unanimously agree that the large quantities of both of these added sugars in soda, sweetened teas, fruit punch, energy drinks, and other sugar-sweetened beverages make them a poor choice for hydration. These beverages provide empty, excess calories.

Carbonated beverages also contain phosphoric acid and artificial colorings. Phosphoric acid is added to cola to give it a tangy flavor, that appealing zing. Not to be confused with the essential mineral phosphorous, phosphoric acid is a chemical additive. Some experts associate high intakes of soda with osteoporosis but cannot pinpoint whether phosphoric acid has anything to do with it.

Caffeine in cola and other caffeinated beverages can interfere with calcium absorption. There is debate as to whether it is the soda itself or the fact that soda has displaced more nutritious beverages, like calcium-rich milk. Soda can also cause stomach upset, gas, and belching, an undesirable effect prior to and during a tennis match.

The merit of cola is the well-supported ergogenic benefit of its caffeine and simple sugar content. Cola has become an increasingly popular "sports drink." A twelve-ounce can of caffeinated cola contains about thirty to forty milligrams of caffeine, about half the amount in an eight-ounce cup of brewed coffee. Despite its sugar content being higher than the desirable carbohydrate profile in sports drinks (One popular brand of cola is 11 percent carbohydrate, while sports drinks range 5–9 percent carbohydrate content), athletes stand by cola for the kick it provides—tennis players included.

The electrifying French tennis star Gaël Monfils caught the media's attention when he poured himself a can of cola during his 2015 Australian Open match against Roger Federer. In a media interview, he claims the elements in cola give him that boost of energy when he is "gassed out." (For further information on the ergogenic benefit of caffeine, refer to chapter 2.)

**Alcoholic Beverages.** A cold beer may be great—for the spectator, not the player! Alcohol can make you feel relaxed at first, relieving the jitters before a big tennis match. However, as it quickly enters the bloodstream, alcohol can make you feel sleepy and groggy. Large amounts of alcohol can cause changes in mood, making it harder to think clearly, focus, and move with coordination—not exactly your performance goal on the tennis court.

Alcohol acts as a depressant. In contrast, caffeine is a stimulant. The physiological impact alcohol has on sports performance contrasts caffeine's influence. Knowing what we know about the established ergogenic benefits of caffeine, alcohol would be the antiergogenic on the tennis court.

Alcoholic beverages also cause the body to lose water, having a diuretic effect—the exact opposite of hydration goals. Many of us have experienced the impact of drinking alcohol through our frequent visits to the bathroom. This causes us to lose excess fluid. Alcohol causes a water shift within the body, giving us the feeling of thirst.[188]

Alcohol also has a lot of calories, seven calories per gram, which is much higher than carbohydrates and protein, each having four calories per gram. One twelve-ounce bottle of regular beer or one five-ounce glass of wine has 150 empty calories with minimal to no nutrition. As little as one drink per day can raise the risk of breast cancer in some women, particularly those who are postmenopausal or who have a family history of breast cancer.[189]

Off the tennis court, are there any merits of moderate alcohol consumption? Research shows that moderate amounts of alcohol may protect healthy adults from developing coronary heart disease. Per the National Institutes of Health, moderation means the following:

No more than one drink per day for women
No more than two drinks per day for men

Women's bodies tend to break down alcohol more slowly, making the risk of impairment in women greater than in men for the same volume of alcohol. Women also have less body water than men, so alcohol can become more concentrated. This is the reason for the differences in alcohol limits between women and men.

One drink equals the following: 12 ounces of regular beer, 5 ounces of wine, and 1.5 ounces of distilled spirits.

Of all alcoholic beverages, red wine has been in the nutritional limelight for quite some time. Red wine is high in the flavonoid antioxidant resveratrol. Animal studies have shown resveratrol to reduce the risk of heart disease by limiting the oxidation of LDL ("bad") cholesterol. Resveratrol has also shown anticancer and anti-inflammatory effects. These results have yet to be demonstrated in humans. Malbec, petite sirah, pinot noir, and cabernet sauvignon are the varieties of red wine containing the highest amount of resveratrol.[190] If you already drink in moderation, red wine may be a better choice than white wine or beer due to its higher antioxidant content.

I have seen many club tennis players drink before, during, and after tennis play. Even though their game is social and fun in nature, this much alcohol consumption could impair judgment enough to run the risk of accidents on and off the court. For those who drink, do so in moderation; for those who do not drink, it is not recommended to start. Drink sensibly, whether on or off the tennis court—or do not drink at all.

# HEAT, HYDRATION AND CHILDREN

Children and teens can practice and play long hours of tennis in the heat. Their energy levels, enthusiasm, and indulgence for sport are admirable, yet these traits can put them at peril of being underhydrated. Combine this with the intensity of all-day junior tennis tournaments, and hydration becomes high priority before, during, and after game day.

There are other hydration considerations unique to children. Juniors are growing and developing, which can influence how their bodies adjust to and regulate themselves in the heat. Children and teens often have erratic eating schedules, eating on the go, balancing school, sports, and other activities. They can have unhealthy diets laden with fast food, salty snacks, and sugary beverages. If these sugary beverages are caffeinated sodas, energy drinks, iced tea, or coffee drinks, the excess amount of caffeine off the court can impact hydration on the court. All these factors compound hydration-related problems in young tennis players.

The American College of Sports Medicine (ACSM) has an excellent summary of hydration in young tennis players. Michael Bergeron, PhD, FACSM (Fellow of the American College of Sports Medicine), executive director at the National Youth Sports Health and Safety Institute, is the foremost expert on hydration in children and teens. In ACSM's *Current Comment* discussion "Heat and Hydration in Young Tennis Players," Bergeron summarizes the special hydration needs for children and teen tennis players.[191]

In recent studies of hydration in teenage boys, Bergeron found that juniors often begin play or training already dehydrated. The more dehydrated the player is at the beginning of a match, the more likely body temperature will rise, affecting both the player's health and tennis performance. Bergeron notes that junior players tend to start a second match more dehydrated than when they began their first match or practice. This makes sense, since there is limited recovery time between the first and second match, and second matches are played later in the day, when it can be much hotter than in the morning.[192] Dehydration (and lack of nutrition) is a key factor in attenuating fatigue in later matches of tournament play.

Children and teens can prevent heat-related hydration performance concerns by hydrating properly before, during, and after exercise. Follow the suggestions below.

**Before the Match.** Too often, nutrition and hydration are thought of on the day of or even a few hours before match or tournament play, when it is too late to fully take advantage of the benefits of a sports nutrition plan. Think at least two to three days ahead of game day to properly plan your fuel and hydration needs. This also gives you confidence, knowing that you are nutritionally primed and hydrated for peak performance.

Drink plenty of fluids ahead of time to ensure you are well hydrated coming into a match. The American College of Sports Medicine suggests that at least four hours before exercise, individuals should drink five to seven milliliters of fluid per kilogram of body weight (two to three milliliters per pound).[193] Using this guideline, a 140-pound female would strive to drink 318–445 milliliters within four hours of her tennis match. This is particularly important if the weather forecast predicts high temperatures and heat index, most often the case in tennis match play. Remember, not drinking enough fluids over a period of time has a cumulative effect. Proper hydration must occur to make up for the fluid deficits from hours and even days earlier. You do not want to make up this fluid "burden" on match day. Drink whether you are thirsty or not.

Acceptable fluids to drink several hours prior to a match, aside from trusty water, include diluted juice, juice, and sports drinks. Stay away from beverages containing large amounts of caffeine or alcohol. Large amounts of caffeine-containing beverages and alcohol act as diuretics, causing you to lose water—not ideal for prematch tennis hydration.

As a gauge to determine if pregame day hydration needs are met, urine should be fairly light colored or almost clear. However, if you are in the bathroom every forty-five minutes or less, you may be drinking too much.[194]

Overhydrating is one of many factors that can lead to hyponatremia. Hyponatremia occurs when the level of sodium in the blood is abnormally low. More common in endurance sports, hyponatremia can still occur in those who overhydrate, especially when they have medical conditions or take prescription drugs that increase risk of hyponatremia. Symptoms of hyponatremia include nausea, vomiting, fatigue, muscle weakness, spasms, and cramping. Note that these symptoms can mimic those of dehydration. You will know if you are overhydrating (versus underhydrating) by the color of your urine, your drinking behavior, and whether you are thirsty or not.[195]

Traveling to play in climates that you are not used to can bring its own set of consequences. Bergeron suggests becoming acclimatized to the climate, particularly hotter weather, seven to ten days prior to your tennis event. If feasible, exercise one to two hours each day in the same heat. Your body will become acclimatized and better adapted to your hydration needs before, during, and after your big match.

**During the Match.** Drink regularly during game day practice and prematch warm-up, particularly when the weather is hot and humid. Once the match starts, drink at every changeover. Tennis play is ideal in this respect. There should never be an excuse for not hydrating during a match.

For match play lasting greater than an hour, sports drinks with water are beneficial. Bergeron and Kovacs suggest drinking 200–240 milliliters of fluid at every changeover.[196] This amount depends on the many factors influencing fluid needs, such as the weather, intensity, and physical demand of the match play and your sweat rate. When the weather is extremely hot (>27° C), fluid needs could be twice this amount.

To replace fluids, sodium, and other electrolytes lost in sweat, use a sports drink. If a sports drink has not quenched thirst or is too "heavy" or tastes too sweet for your palate, use a combination of sports drink and water until thirst is relieved.

Hydrate throughout the match, no matter what the score or how long or short the match goes. Do not let a match score dictate your hydration decision making. Who would not savor a favorable changeover match score of 6–1, 5–2? A score like this can make us become overconfident and underfocused, causing us to relax our hydration habits in favor of thinking about our weekend plans. This subtle letdown can affect our performance, both physically and mentally. When the opponent is fighting for every point, while we have relaxed our behaviors, match tide can turn. This reversal of fortune can lead to a demanding third set or a match-deciding tiebreaker—when hydration and nutrition are still critically important.

**After the Match.** The goal is to fully replace any fluid and electrolyte deficit after tennis. If another match is played the same day or even the following day, it is essential to adequately restore fluids and electrolytes to normal balance. After the final match of the day, sodium and potassium can be replenished in postmatch foods through normal meals and snacks. Drinking water or fluids with nutrients will hydrate during meal time and thereafter. If schedules do not permit a full meal or snack, sports drinks can more conveniently replace fluids and electrolytes.[197]

For rapid and complete fluid recovery during tennis played in hot, humid climate, drink 1.5 liters (50.7 ounces) of fluid for each kilogram of body weight lost.[198] As an example, one kilogram, or 2.2 pounds, lost would equal three liters of post-tennis fluid replacement. Bergeron suggests drinking 150 percent of fluid deficit after play. This means for every pound lost from tennis play, drink an additional twenty-four ounces, or another 730 milliliters.[199] This is especially important in tournaments, when another match is played later in the afternoon, most often in hotter weather than the first match.

Make every attempt to drink fluids over time rather than guzzling large amounts all at once. Drinking fluids rapidly will cause increased urine production, which will cause you to lose fluids more quickly. Drinking recovery fluids slowly, over time, will cause you to retain them better by minimizing excess trips to the bathroom. At every stage of hydration, refer to the urine color chart to assess whether fluid needs have been met.

The American College of Sports Medicine summarizes hydration recommendations before, during and after exercise in table 7.4.[200]

**Table 7.4: Fluids Before, During, and After Exercise (Source: ACSM)**

| | How Much | What to Drink |
|---|---|---|
| **Before Exercise** (Four hours prior) | 2–3 ml per pound | Water or sports drink |
| **During Exercise** | Very dependent on sweat rate, climate, intensity, and duration of tennis. In general, 120–240 ml for every fifteen minutes of exercise | Water and sports drink |
| **After Exercise** | 1.5 L per kilogram of body weight lost | Water and sports drink |

Both children and adult tennis players need to make hydration a top priority. Good hydration is essential for both tournament and single match play that can go the distance on a hot, blistery court. Hydration planning includes choosing the right kind and amount of fluids. Introduced early in this chapter, Marcus learned to never again rely on energy drinks for his hydration needs. He still enjoys his favorite energy drink for an afternoon kick at work, but water and sports drinks have become his ally on the tennis court.

# 8

# NUTRITION BAG CHECK: SNACKS FOR TENNIS PERFORMANCE

**Be bold. If you're going to make an error, make a doozy and don't be afraid to hit the ball.**
—Billie Jean King

Tracy enjoys playing competitive singles for her 4.0 USTA team. She thrives on pressure, eking out many close tiebreak matches with her mental toughness, perseverance, and fitness level. Tracy met her match when one of her opponents, a former collegiate basketball player (needless to say, an exceptional athlete), took her to the distance in her team-deciding court number-one singles match. Playing in the steamy Arizona weather in late May, Tracy rallied and lost a close and long first set 6–7. She soon felt dizzy and light-headed; the changeover could not happen soon enough. She plunked herself down on the player's bench. Desperately reaching for a snack in her voluminous tennis bag, she awkwardly groped each pocket, becoming frantic when nothing edible materialized. Tracy's teammate quickly got her a sports drink, banana, and sports beans from her own tennis bag stash before Tracy passed out. Tracy immediately felt better. She had run out of fuel, with glycogen stores diminished and blood sugar dropping. Grateful to have her friend provide her energy relief, Tracy fought hard but lost her match in a three-hour battle she had not anticipated.

## FUELING DURING TENNIS PLAY

Understanding the importance of carbohydrates, leaving your tennis bag devoid of a healthy snack would be nutritional negligence. Since a match can last an unpredictable one, two, or three hours, be sure to have adequate fuel in your tennis bag to restore your glycogen stores and satisfy hunger. You also ensure your body gets the nutrition it needs when you miss that meal during your marathon match.

When strenuous exercise lasts more than sixty minutes, athletes need carbohydrates to replenish glycogen stores. This should amount to thirty to sixty grams of carbohydrate for exercise lasting more than one hour. Eating a healthy snack during a long tennis match also curbs hunger pangs. Snacks should be easy to chew and digest, so their nutrients are quickly absorbed and utilized. Always have an appetizing snack that works for you in your tennis bag.

A healthy snack boosts the nutrition in your diet, on or off the court. But what should you pull from your tennis bag for the fuel you need during a grueling match? Pretzels, a candy bar, a protein bar, or the trusty banana?

Before answering this question, one caveat always prevails: if it works for you, stick with it. If you are convinced your favorite tennis bag snack produces winning results, stay with it. Tennis is a mental game. If superstitious regimen, including food selection, helps build your confidence, go for it!

Of the above examples, the snack that should not belong

in your tennis bag is a candy bar. Candy bars are high in fat, containing palm kernel oil, a type of saturated fat, as well as refined sugar. High-fat, high-sugar snacks—like cookies, candy bars, and brownies—take time for your body to digest. This also applies to high-fat, salty snacks like potato chips and corn chips. Although the sodium in chips may be beneficial to replace sweat losses, the high fat content should stay out of your tennis bag during match play.

From recreational beginners to professional superstars, many tennis players turn to candy bars to satisfy their hunger and fuel their game. Prior to making his diet transformation, Novak Djokovic, one of the greatest players of our time, describes his routine eating pattern. In his book *Serve to Win: The 14-Day Gluten-free Plan for Physical and Mental Excellence*, Djokovic writes,

> I was heavy, slow and tired because I was eating the way most of us eat. I ate like a Serb (and an American)—plenty of Italian food like pizza, pasta, and especially bread as well as heavy meat dishes at least a couple of times a day. I snacked on candy bars and other sugary foods during matches, thinking they would help to keep my energy up and figured my training schedule had earned me a handful off every cookie tray that passed by.[201]

Most recently, tennis pro and former number-six men's player in the world, Gilles Simon, requested a chocolate candy bar from the match referee during the 2015 Australian Open against countryman Gaël Monfils.

Fats in mixed meals and candy bars slow down the time their carbohydrates digest and convert to glucose. Glucose fuels the muscles and brain. Although candy bars fill you up and satisfy hunger, the delay in gastric, or stomach, emptying diverts the needed energy from thirsty muscles to digestion. This may cause you to feel heavy and sluggish—the exact opposite of the nimble agility you want to have on the court. These snacks are also low in nutrition. Reserve these snacks for an occasional treat after you complete your tennis match, not during it.

Protein bars are a good choice for postmatch snack recovery but not the ideal choice during match play. Protein bars can be deceiving. What looks like a perfectly healthy ergogenic aid could be a glorified candy bar in disguise, laden with fat, sugar, and additives. Many brands fill a good percentage of their total fat content with saturated and trans fats. Some protein bars can have half their calories coming from fat.

Protein and fat take longer for the body to digest. During match play, muscles need fast-acting carbohydrates for fuel. A good-quality protein bar is excellent as a postworkout recovery food. After exercise, protein bars replenish muscle amino acids, provide calories and nutrition, and satisfy hunger.

With so many protein bars on the market, what should you look for? If your protein bar is a post-tennis recovery snack, look for a bar that is modest in calories (around 250 calories or fewer) and not a meal replacement bar (e.g., 400 calories). Be sure to read labels, and select a protein bar that has minimal saturated and trans fat, simple sugars, and processed ingredients. A short ingredient listing is a good sign your protein bar is not full of unwanted, unneeded additives. Get your protein from whey protein. Recent research gives the edge to whey protein in its muscle-building effect compared to soy protein.[202] If you are vegan, protein from soy, peas, or brown rice are good options. Look for a bar that has whole ingredients, such as whole grain, nuts, and dried fruit; is minimally processed; and tastes good.

Can't find the ideal protein bar? You can build your own protein bar by choosing ingredients from www.youbars.com. This website will provide nutritional analysis, packaging, and shipping of your very own custom protein bar. You even choose the name of your protein bar.

Although a good-quality protein bar is great for post-tennis recovery, the best during-match play snacks deliver carbohydrates to fuel muscles for those deep, winning ground strokes and crisp volleys. Pretzels and bananas both contain carbohydrates. Both are excellent during-match snacks. The carbohydrate in bananas is from starch and the naturally occurring simple sugar fructose. Starch and fructose take longer to digest and convert to glucose than foods containing sucrose, glucose, or maltodextrin. If your goal is to have an immediate energy boost, then pretzels chased with a sports drink would accomplish this.

If your goal is to fulfill hunger pangs while still getting a healthy dose of carbs for sustained energy, bananas are always a great choice for tennis players. Bananas come in their own convenient packaging, which makes them an easy snack to transport in a tennis bag. Bananas are also high in potassium. Like sodium, potassium is an electrolyte that needs to be replenished due to sweat loss. Tennis players battling in a hot, humid climate know all too well the copious amount of sweat loss that can occur during a match. Potassium regulates fluid balance and stabilizes controlled and automatic muscle contractions.

In addition to potassium, bananas also contain other important nutrients. One medium banana provides 25 percent of the RDA for vitamin B6. Vitamin B6, or pyridoxine, is one of the B-complex vitamins required to help convert food into energy. Bananas also contain vitamin C, manganese, biotin, copper, prebiotics, and fiber. With all this good nutrition, many experts consider bananas to be the perfect ergogenic snack.

One banana has about three grams of soluble fiber. Soluble fiber absorbs water and swells up into a gel-like substance. By doing so, soluble fiber slows digestion and prevents absorption of cholesterol. Instead of entering our bloodstream, the soluble fiber in bananas and other foods, like beans and oatmeal, cause cholesterol to be eliminated from our bodies.

Singing the praises of the banana, why would there be debate about the effectiveness of this reliable standby for tennis fuel? Bananas contain both simple carbohydrates and starch. Starch tends to take longer for the body to digest and turn into glucose for fuel. If this is an on-court concern, couple a banana with the fast-acting carbs in a sports drink. The starch from a banana will help sustain blood glucose; the carbs from the sports drink will quickly deliver energy to tired muscles. On the tennis court, bananas are a much better choice than a candy bar.

A brown-spotted banana is sweeter than a green one. A ripe banana (or any ripe fruit) contains a higher amount of total carbohydrate and simple sugars compared to a green, unripe banana. Green, unripe bananas contain more starch. Be sure to have a bright-yellow banana in your tennis bag to get the benefit of both sugar and starch.

Studies show that getting a variety of carbs from various food and fluid sources for both quick and sustained energy is ideal for working muscles.[203] Combining a sports drink containing dextrose (and sucrose) with a banana containing starch and fructose is a perfect example of combining a variety of carbohydrate sources for exercise fuel.

I have selected the top ten snacks for your tennis bag for several reasons. All provide fast-acting carbohydrates as well as other nutrients, including vitamins, minerals, and phytonutrients. They are easy to carry and are nonperishable. Many tennis players find these snacks delicious and easy to digest.

The specific portion size of each match snack provides approximately twenty-five to thirty grams of carbohydrates. If strenuous tennis play lasts more than sixty minutes, add twenty ounces of sports drink for thirty grams of fast-acting carbohydrates every additional hour of play. This is in addition to your healthy snack. Keep nonperishable carbohydrate snacks in your tennis bag at all times.

Remember, these snacks replenish carbohydrates during exercise. If athletes have not started out with a full supply of glycogen, their carbohydrate reserves will quickly be used. Additional carbohydrate will be needed to "catch up" or make up for this depletion. Always plan your diet hours and days ahead of your tournament or match to ensure you have a full supply of glycogen to fuel those winning volleys.

## TOP TEN SNACKS TO PACK IN YOUR TENNIS BAG

1. **Grapes** (about thirty medium green or red seedless grapes, which fit in one cup) get quickly digested and readily converted to glucose or fuel for muscles and brain. Grapes contain the sugars, glucose, and fructose. Count them out once, and then you will have an idea of the portion equivalent to thirty grams of carbohydrate— approximately one cup of grapes.

2. **Pretzels** (one ounce, or twenty minipretzels) provide carbs and sodium. Chew well to break down carbohydrates. Pretzels can be dry, so make sure to drink a sports drink or water to help chew, swallow, digest, and absorb their valuable carbohydrates. Pretzels also contain salt, or sodium chloride. Sodium and chloride are two minerals lost in sweat. Eating salted pretzels replaces these essential minerals. One ounce of pretzels contains approximately 250 milligrams of sodium.

3. **Raisins** (one small, 1.5-ounce box) contain carbohydrates, potassium, fiber, and iron. Be sure to chew raisins well. Raisins and other dried fruits can be hard to digest and could cause an upset stomach. If this is the case, select a snack that is easier to digest.

4. **Granola bars** are convenient to carry in a tennis bag, do not easily spoil, and contain whole grain, carbs, and B vitamins. One small, chewy granola bar contains about

twenty grams of carbohydrate. Chew well and wash down with water or sports drink to aid digestion and absorption.

5. **Cereal bars** are also convenient, having the advantage of containing fortified cereal, which provides extra vitamins and minerals. One cereal bar contains about twenty-five grams of carbohydrate, mostly from whole grains and natural sugars from fruit. Combine with water or a sports drink to facilitate digestion and absorption.

6. **Bananas** (one large) are nature's conveniently wrapped snack, containing carbohydrates, potassium, manganese, vitamin B6, vitamin C, and soluble fiber. It is no wonder bananas are the tennis player's ideal snack choice. Bananas contain a combination of carbohydrates from starch and the simple sugar fructose. One large banana contains the perfect dose of thirty grams of carbohydrate. To curb hunger pangs during long matches, bananas provide satiety with their starch content while still providing needed sugars. A riper banana will contain more simple sugars than starch. Sweeter, riper bananas have a higher glycemic index than unripe bananas.

7. **Rice cakes** are light and easy to digest. Rice cakes have a high glycemic index, their carbohydrates quickly converting to glucose. Today's rice cakes come in a variety of blends and flavors, including rye, corn, and brown rice. Rice cakes are very low in calories, fat, and sodium, unlike many other snack chips and crackers. They are gluten-free. Four rice cakes (nine grams each) contain about 140 calories and thirty grams of carbohydrate.

8. **Crackers.** Wheat crackers, Goldfish crackers, and saltines provide carbohydrates, sodium and B vitamins. Crackers made with refined flour have a higher glycemic index compared to whole-grains crackers. Whole-grain crackers are higher in fiber. Avoid high-fiber crackers if they are hard for you to digest during a match. Also, steer clear of

crackers if hydrogenated fats high in artificial trans fats are tops in their ingredient listing.

9. **Cereal mix** made with fortified cereal plus additional carbs from pretzels and crackers is another option. One cup of cereal mix contains about thirty grams of carbohydrates. You can make your own mix using rice and corn cereals for a healthy, gluten-free tennis snack.

10. **Cereal** is not just for breakfast. Even though a small baggie of cereal may not be the most exciting snack to pack, the nutrition in dry cereal is hard to beat. Almost everyone has a box of cereal in their cupboard. Cereals like toasted Os, Chex, corn puffs, and corn flakes provide fast-acting carbohydrates with added vitamins and minerals. Be wary of high-fiber, low-glycemic-index cereals, which take longer to digest and absorb. Make sure to reserve these healthy whole-grain cereals for breakfast or off-court snacking. There are about thirty grams of carbohydrate in two-thirds to three-quarters of a cup of cereal. Wash down cereal with water or sports drink for faster digestion and absorption of nutrients.

You may notice that almonds (or any kind of nut) are missing from the list of tennis bag snacks. Nuts are excellent sources of unsaturated fat and protein. But remember, the goal of tennis snacks is to provide fuel during tennis and satisfy hunger. Although the fat and protein in almonds satisfies hunger, almonds contain no carbohydrates for quick fuel. All their calories come from fat and protein.

Although various trail mixes contain carbohydrates from oats, seeds, and dried fruit, they may also contain nuts and chocolate, carob, peanut butter, or yogurt chips, which provide protein and fat. Like protein bars, nuts and trail mix are excellent for postmatch recovery but not ideal during a match when quickly digestible, fast-acting carbohydrates are essential for sustained tennis performance.

Snacking on and off the court can be a nutritious supplement to your diet. For elite athletes, snacking is necessary to achieve the high number of calories needed for athletic performance. Be wise about snack selection. For off-court snacking, have these healthy snacks in your cooler, backpack, locker, desk drawer, kitchen cupboard, and refrigerator—wherever you can reach for them when a snack attack hits. Snacks are divided into their most predominant macronutrient: carbohydrates, protein, or fat. Many of these snacks, like nuts, have both protein and fat, offering the goodness of a variety of nutrition.

## SNACKING FOR HIGH ENERGY NUTRITION

### CARBOHYDRATES:
Fruit: fresh, dried, frozen (canned, if the first three are not accessible)
Cut vegetables (pair with hummus, dip, guacamole)
Cereal: cold cereal, granola, oatmeal
Whole-grain crackers
Whole-grain and multigrain chips: brown rice, amaranth, corn
Baked chips: sweet potato or white potato
Chips: fried in canola or olive oil
Popcorn
Trail mix
Whole-grain breads: bagels, homemade muffins, bread/toast
Cereal bars
Breakfast biscuit or cookie
Granola bars

### PROTEIN:
Nut butters: peanut, almond, cashew
Greek yogurt, yogurt

Protein smoothies
Protein bars
Hummus
Bean dip
Quinoa salad
Canned tuna, canned salmon
Cheese sticks
Cheese

**FAT:**
Avocado slices
Guacamole
Nuts: walnuts, almonds, cashews, peanuts, pecans, macadamia nuts, pistachios, brazil nuts, pine nuts
Soy nuts
Seeds: hemp, chia, flax, sesame, sunflower, pumpkin

Let's revisit Tracy from the beginning of the chapter. Normally always prepared for a match, the one time she forgot to pack snacks in her tennis bag was the match she lost. She attributed the loss to fatigue resulting from lack of fuel for high-energy tennis play. Since this unpleasant experience, Tracy always packs a healthy snack in her tennis bag.

# 9

# TENNIS NUTRITION FOR CHILDREN AND TEENS

**Good, better, best. May you never rest until your good is better and your better is best.**
—Anonymous

Gabriel is a seventeen-year-old senior in high school and aspiring collegiate player. He stands five foot eleven and weighs 130 pounds. He needs to gain weight and muscle mass to compete with the larger, fitter players. Gabriel says he knows the players who eat well are the ones who'll win. Between tennis practice and working out in the gym, he needs to consume upward of four thousand calories each day to reach his weight goal of 160 pounds. The challenge is that Gabriel just doesn't like to eat. He is a self-proclaimed "eat to live," not "live to eat" eater. His diet includes typical teen favorites, from pizza to toaster pastries, always a soda within arm's reach. He knows from firsthand experience that these types of foods adversely affect his tennis fitness and performance. He complains of fatigue and lack of energy on and off the court. Like many teenagers on the go, Gabriel wants to know what he can eat to gain weight and supercharge his fitness to propel his game to the next level.

## NUTRITION CHALLENGES FOR TENNIS KIDS

Who would be better to discuss the challenges tennis kids face than Steve Smith? He is the inspirational tennis coach who has fostered the successful development of children and teens—many of whom have become collegiate and professional stars. Smith has coached twelve collegiate students who have won NCAA National Championships. Smith developed the first ever college accredited curriculum and degree plan designed to teach the game of tennis.

Smith believes that in order for children to become world-class players, they need to start making healthy food and beverage choices early in their childhoods. Then, by high school and college, they are as fit as their world-class tennis competition.[204] It's not too late for adults either. Smith identifies a number of tennis legends who changed their diets during their career and saw winning results, including legends Martina Navratilova and Pete Sampras.

Smith understands that children and teens struggle to make healthy food and beverage choices. With our American lifestyle characterized by fast food and sugary beverages, portion distortion, eating on the run, and television, cell phones, computers, and gaming devices literally at the dinner table, healthy eating seems elusive.[205] With American culture evolving and changing, so too have our children's diet and exercise habits. Nick Bollettieri concurs insofar as declaring that lack of proper nutrition is the greatest detriment to the health of children and adults—worldwide.[206]

A former tennis professional I know, who is now a tennis coach in Sarasota, Florida, asks his young tennis players what they have eaten before their match or drilling session. One of his female prodigies shared her menu with me: chips and salsa for breakfast, a skipped lunch, and a large burrito with extra hot sauce for dinner. She added that she loved to play on the Xbox in her free time. Obviously, this regimen is not a winning fitness combination.

We all know children and teens have an affinity for certain foods that tend to be high in fat and sugar and low in nutrition. Surprisingly, the amount of empty calories children consume from foods containing solid fats and sugars has declined from 1994 to 2010 and most recently leveled off.[207] However, the intake of these empty calories continues to exceed the discretionary allowance suggested by health professionals. Reedy and Krebs-Smith listed the following top sources of added fats and sugars in children and teens:

1. Grain desserts, such as cakes, cookies, doughnuts, pastries
2. Pizza
3. Sugar-sweetened beverages, which include soda plus sugary fruit drinks; calories from sugar-sweetened beverages alone were high enough to use up the discretionary limit for empty calories for the entire day[208]

There are more convenient, processed, and fast foods readily available for eating on the go outside of the home than ever before. Especially appealing to children and teens, these foods tend to be calorie dense, sweet, fatty, salty, or all the above. In addition, the low cost, large portions, and drive-through convenience of fast foods make supersized sodas and french fries hard to resist.

This drive-by eating translates into an astounding number of excess calories with consequences. Consistently choosing these salty, high-fat, high-sugar, nutrient-poor foods over more nutritious ones becomes deleterious to our health. Coupled with a lack of activity, the state of children's nutritional health and weight status is troubling.

Currently, 32 percent of American children are classified as overweight or obese. The CDC predicts that one in three American children born in 2000 will develop diabetes as a result of obesity.[209] Children under the age of ten are already developing type 2 diabetes, a disease primarily seen in adults over the age of forty.

Overweight and obesity can take an emotional toll on children. They continue to carry a social stigma (even though two-thirds of Americans are overweight or obese). Overweight children and teens may struggle with their body image and self-esteem. In a worst-case scenario, being picked on or bullied can lead to emotional trauma and eating disorders in children and teens.

How can parents foster healthy eating in their child athlete? I recently attended an outstanding seminar sponsored by the Institute of Natural Resources entitled "Food Habits, Cravings and Emotions." Michelle Albers, PhD, RD, identified the dos and don'ts of emotional overeating in children. These tips help cultivate healthy eating behaviors.[210] Parents, coaches, and teachers should pay heed to these suggestions, as they teach children the foundation of good eating habits.

### Dos

- Tell the child to listen to his or her internal cues about hunger, eating, and fullness.
- Encourage the child to eat in response to his/her physical hunger and to stop eating when feeling full.
- Encourage the child to eat more slowly and really enjoy his or her food.
- Expose and provide a wide variety of all types of food to the child.
- Encourage physical activity for pleasure (e.g., "Let's play tennis or go for a jog on the beach").
- Help the child find ways to deal with emotions and boredom in ways other than reaching for food. Reading, taking a walk or a bike ride, or playing a pickup basketball game at the park are good examples.
- Help the child understand there is more to life than food, weight, and trying to obtain the "perfect body."

- Compliment attributes like integrity, kindness, and creativity rather than physical attributes like body size, weight, or shape.

## Don'ts

- Don't use food as a reward for good behavior. Giving candy or treats for positive reinforcement or recognition is a no-no. Compliments and praise, not candy bars, build self-esteem.
- Don't tell the child that eating certain foods will make him or her feel better. Talk to your child about what's getting him or her down. A bowl of ice cream is only a pacifier.
- Don't use food as guilt (e.g., "Eat all your food; children are starving in the world").
- Don't deny certain desirable foods for bad or undesirable behavior (e.g., "We are not getting pizza if you don't win your match").
- Don't make the child eat certain things to get what they want (e.g., "If you eat your vegetables, I will buy you those jeans").
- Don't coax the child to eat foods he or she does not want.
- Don't forbid any foods, such as sweets (e.g., "No chocolate for a week if you don't get an A on your test").
- Don't significantly restrict the amounts of food the child eats. Children are growing and developing. Unless advised by a physician, a child's calories should not be restricted, especially for an active tennis player.
- Don't overemphasize an ideal beauty or body shape. Children are impressionable, especially when it comes to cultural images of beauty, thinness, or body build.
- Don't criticize the child's body size, shape, or type.
- Don't speak negatively about your own body size and shape.

- Don't claim that a particular diet, weight, or body size will automatically lead to happiness and fulfillment.
- Don't promote dieting behavior. Children model parental behavior. If parents are constantly on diets or even do them together with their children, they may send the wrong message about healthy eating.[211]

With planning, self-discipline, and parental support, good nutrition can become a daily reality to young children. While coaches can teach strokes, serves, and strategy, parents teach nutrition by setting a good example for their young children early on in the home. Once children become teens and can make independent choices, they should have the nutritional knowledge base to make wise food decisions. Of course, not every food or beverage choice a child or teen makes will be ideal. However, having the tools to make well-thought-out decisions about food and nutrition is critical in helping children become healthy adults.

Like adults, children need adequate nutrition, both macronutrients (protein, carbohydrates, and fat) and micronutrients (vitamins and minerals), as well as fluids and fiber to promote health and optimize tennis performance. The distinct difference in nutrient needs between children and adults is that children are growing and developing while undergoing an often rigorous tennis training program.

As a result, calorie or energy needs for children are significantly higher than for adults based on their body weight, body surface area, and the fact they are rapidly growing and developing. During the life span, children require the most calories, and then adolescents, and then adults. Intense tennis training necessitates substantially more calories to fuel an active child's or teen's day.

As with calories, children need a higher amount of protein per body weight to ensure normal growth and development as compared to adults. Adequate protein during childhood builds muscle tissue, bones, organs, and hormones. Do child athletes need more protein than their inactive counterparts? Research is unclear about whether children need more protein for optimal performance beyond that needed for growth and development.[212] In fact, there is minimal research done on sports nutrition for children.

Children eating a Western diet tend to get more than adequate protein. Special consideration needs to be given in certain situations. If children are self-restricting calories in attempt to lose weight to enhance sports performance, protein as well as other nutrients may fall short of needs. Children who are on vegan, gluten-free, diabetic, or other diets may have more challenges getting adequate nutrients, including protein. Children and teens who restrict calories, have multiple food allergies or intolerances, and/or follow special diets would benefit with the help of a CSSD or RD.

By all means, if a child or teen has an eating disorder, parents, friends, teachers, and coaches must seek medical attention for him or her. This early support helps ensure children and teens meet their nutritional needs for normal growth and development and addresses the psychosocial issues that come with eating disorders.

Bob Davis provides his insights on childhood obesity. This accomplished tennis pro was junior doubles partner with the legendary Arthur Ashe. As inductee and president of the Black Tennis Hall of Fame, Davis heads the Panda Foundation, an organization whose mission is to address childhood obesity through nutrition, fitness, and self-respect. I have the privilege of working with Davis's foundation as nutrition educator. Volunteers working with Davis's organization teach after-school tennis as a means of getting children hooked on tennis and physical activity.

Davis firmly believes that nutrition education will only be effective if parents model what their children are taught. In other words, children's eating behaviors will not change if parents continue to, in effect, serve unhealthy food at the dinner table or be uninvolved with nutrition in the home. Children will change their eating behaviors if they have positive role models in the home who put good nutrition in practice from the market to the kitchen table.[213]

## NUTRITION TIPS FOR TENNIS PARENTS AND COACHES

Parents can encourage sound diet and nutrition habits using the tips below. Coaches are influential too. The ITF and USTA provide valuable coach mentoring programs. Diet, nutrition, and hydration are several of many topics in their coaching curriculum. When children follow suit, good nutrition practices can give them that winning tennis edge.

1. **Eat breakfast—and eat a healthy one.** Breakfast is the one meal that children and teens can prepare and manage early in the morning. Children need to make breakfast a priority as they do other morning rituals, like brushing teeth and taking a shower. Breakfast meals should provide one-third of the day's nutritional goal. Specific nutrients in many common breakfast foods include vitamin C, folic acid, iron, calcium, and fiber. All this nutritional goodness equates to a glass of orange juice and a bowl of cereal with milk. It's that simple. Breakfast can be very easy for children and teens, even when the family is rushing to get ready for work or school.

    Eating breakfast provides clear benefits to children. Studies show that children who eat breakfast are more alert and focused in the classroom.[214] Breakfast provides an opportunity for families to eat together. Busy as the morning rush can be, simple-to-prepare breakfasts can make a few minutes of family dining at the table more feasible. Take a new look at these simple, healthy breakfast mainstays, perfect for children and teens on the go:

- whole-grain cereal with milk and sliced banana or fresh berries
- whole-grain toast with peanut butter
- toasted bagel with avocado, tomato, and spinach leaves
- oatmeal with dried fruit, crushed flaxseed, and nuts
- scrambled or boiled egg with english muffin
- frozen waffle or pancake with sliced bananas, walnuts, and syrup
- greek yogurt with piece of fresh fruit and a granola bar
- breakfast cereal bar and a piece of fruit
- yogurt smoothie with your favorite fresh fruit, vegetables, and nuts
- sliced apples with peanut butter and a small box of raisins
- cottage cheese and peaches with a cereal bar
- breakfast quesadilla with scrambled egg, cheese, and salsa
- peanut-butter-and-all-fruit-jelly sandwich
- individual trail mix baggy with an eight-ounce yogurt

Include a calcium-rich beverage, such as calcium-fortified orange juice, soy, almond, coconut, skim, or low-fat milk or yogurt drink, and the above breakfast meals provide the energy, nutrients, and satiety for children to perform at their peak—both physically and academically.

2. **Eat a healthy lunch.** Children have two options for lunch: a packed lunch from home or school lunch from the cafeteria. While tater tots and hot dogs may still be

around, schools now provide salad bars, bottled water, skim milk, veggie burgers, and baked fries.

The federal National School Lunch Program has been in public schools since 1947. Times have since changed. In 2010, the landmark Healthy, Hunger-Free Kids Act was passed—its mission to address childhood obesity and improve nutrition.

This act requires schools to increase the availability of fruits, vegetables, and whole grains in meals and snacks while reducing saturated fat, trans fats, sugar, and sodium. The act also requires school food service programs to set calorie limits for age appropriateness—in other words, adjusting portions sizes and calories based on age groups: smaller bodies, smaller calories; larger bodies, larger calories.[215]

Many schools have voluntarily removed salty, high-fat snacks and regular soda from vending machines. The 2010 Smart Snacks in School proposal creates a national standard for healthy food and beverage offerings. Starting in school year 2014/2015, the Smart Snacks in School regulation requires that all food sold in school, including at the school store and in vending machines, meet nutrition standards. This act promotes snacks with low-fat dairy, whole grains, and fruits and vegetables as their main ingredient, not added refined sugars and trans fats.[216]

Parents can assist children in making good school lunch choices. They can post the school lunch menu on the refrigerator and discuss healthy choices with their child. Many school menus identify the day's healthy choices in an easy-to-understand format for kids and parents. Some schools make nutritional breakdowns for their menus available on websites and in newsletters. Many school food service programs utilize RDs for menu planning, nutrition advocacy, and wellness education.

For the parents and children who prefer to brown-bag it from home, be sure to plan wisely. A packed lunch should not only satisfy hunger and appetite but also provide at least a quarter of the day's nutrient intake. Getting nutrients from packed lunches only works when the lunch is eaten. Making the lunchbox lunch appetizing is important. Keep your kids from trading their tuna sandwiches for their buddy's chocolate chip cookies by balancing appeal with nutrition.

Accompany a healthy packed lunch with a nutritious beverage. Options include water, 100 percent fruit juice, and shelf-stable individual soy milk boxes. Always keep milk as an option. Standing in line for the nutrition in a half pint of skim or 1 percent milk is worth the wait. Here are some nutrition-powered lunchbox ideas you or your child can pack:

- peanut-butter-and-jelly sandwich on whole-grain bread with an apple and yogurt smoothie; try all-natural peanut or almond butter and an all-fruit, no-added-sugar fruit spread
- turkey and swiss cheese on bagel or sandwich pocket with lettuce or spinach leaves and tomato, veggie chips, and grapes
- chili (leftover from dinner) with whole-wheat crackers, orange, and homemade cornbread
- tomato soup, string cheese, pretzels, and oatmeal-raisin cookies
- roast beef on rye bread and olive oil mayo with mandarin orange cup and multigrain chips

- chicken Caesar wrap (homemade or premade from the market), black-bean tortilla chips with hummus, and strawberries
- leftover spaghetti with meat sauce (made with lean beef, ground turkey, tofu crumbles, or tempeh), fresh pear, and two small dark chocolate squares

3. **Eat the family meal together.** Many readers may recall ritual family dinners with table gingerly set and a homemade, hot meal from scratch—images of a dinner bell ringing at 5:00 p.m. sharp. With today's changing family dynamic, eating dinner together can be challenging. With parents working and children in after-school activities, just getting to eat dinner before bedtime is a feat in and of itself for busy families.

Research demonstrates the benefits of eating family meals together. Evidence supports a positive association between the frequency of family meals and quality of diet in teens. In a review of studies examining the frequency of shared family meals in relation to nutritional health, Amber Hammons, PhD, found that children and teens who share family meals three or more times a week are more likely to be in a normal weight range and have healthier eating habits than those who share fewer than three meals together. They were also less likely to have disordered eating.[217] A recent study led by Nicole Larson, PhD, MPH, RD, showed that eating family breakfast together was associated with higher intake of fruits, whole grain, and fiber, as well as a lower risk of overweight/obesity in teenagers.[218]

Parents can encourage healthy, nutritious eating when they eat with their children at the dinner table. Family mealtime also promotes undivided time for dialogue and communication—an opportunity that rarely comes up during the hub of a busy day.

4. **Hydrate with water or fluids with nutrition.** Some experts feel sugar-sweetened beverages are the culprit promoting overweight and obesity in children (and adults). From regular soda and sugary fruit drinks to caffeine-laden energy drinks and teas, children are overwhelmed with colorful, appealing sugar-sweetened beverages, many directly marketed to teens and young adults. While total fat intake has declined over the years, carbohydrate intake from added sugars in food and drink has increased, contributing empty calories with minimal nutrition.

Portion distortion also makes its presence known in these high-calorie beverages. Fast-food restaurants supersize their drinks; convenience stores promote deals on forty-eight-ounce sodas; and most beverage manufacturers' average-sized bottled sodas top twenty ounces, the equivalent of sixteen teaspoons of sugar! It's no wonder children are drinking a large number of empty calories from these beverages. They would be much better off drinking calorie-free water or fluids with nutrition, such as milk or 100 percent fruit juice.

Promote healthy beverage selections early on in the home. Take every measure to keep soda and sugary fruit drinks out of the house, making water, 100 percent juice, and skim, 1 percent, and fortified almond, rice, or soy milk available. Encourage sports drinks for the gym or tennis court, not at the dinner table. Sports drinks replenish fluids, sodium, potassium, and carbohydrates during prolonged exercise—what they were engineered to do. Otherwise, they only add extra sugar, sodium, and calories at the dinner table.

# THE CALCIUM SHORTFALL IN CHILDREN

Children require calcium, phosphorous, and vitamin D to support rapid bone growth and development in the childhood and teen years. The teen years are the most crucial bone-building years for both boys and girls. Calcium and vitamin D help mineralize or build bone during the childhood years. This process is completed by the end of the teenage years.

The United States has seen a decline in children's milk intake, creating a shortfall of necessary calcium in these critical years. The calcium requirement for children ages nine through eighteen is 1,300 milligrams per day, the highest of any stage of life. In a 2010 evaluation, the National Health and Examination Survey, which evaluates the dietary adequacy of Americans, found that calcium was well below the RDA for girls and boys aged nine through thirteen and teenage girls aged fourteen through eighteen, who were getting less than 700 milligrams per day.[219] Calcium intake is especially important in girls, who will later experience calcium-related bone loss in their child-bearing years and menopause.

To add to this calcium shortfall, lifestyle choices—such as smoking and alcohol and caffeine consumption—can limit the absorption of calcium. In most households, sugary beverages, sports drinks, and soda have replaced calcium-rich beverages at meal and snack times. Table 9.1 lists calcium requirement in children.

**Table 9.1: Calcium Recommendations for Children and Teens (Source: Food and Nutrition Board, Institute of Medicine)**

| Age (years) | Calcium Requirement (mg) |
|---|---|
| 1–3 | 700 |
| 4–8 | 1,000 |
| 9–18 | 1,300 |

Calcium needs can be met by two to four servings of low-fat dairy products per day, including yogurt, milk, and cheese. Nondairy sources, such as calcium-fortified orange juice and almond, rice, hemp, coconut, and soy milk, are also high in calcium. With the availability of so many milks on grocery store shelves, there should be no reason these calcium-rich options would be in short supply (chapter 1 lists food and beverage sources of calcium).

## GETTING CHILDREN AND TEENS TO GET ENOUGH CALCIUM AND VITAMIN D, TODAY'S CHALLENGE:

### TEENS AND CHILDREN THINK DAIRY PRODUCTS ARE FATTENING

Teens, especially adolescent girls, may think that dairy products are high in calories. This is a misconception. Whole milk or full-fat dairy products are higher in calories and saturated fat than low-fat or fat-free dairy products. Low-fat or fat-free dairy products provide potent nutrition with very few calories.

Although studies are inconclusive, University of Tennessee research showed that people who routinely include low-fat or fat-free dairy products in a healthy diet weigh less than those who do not.[220] Various theories abound on why drinking milk could cause weight loss or maintenance (or could not).[221] It is possible that substituting high-protein, calcium-rich milk for unhealthy beverages like soda can cause a feeling of fullness or satiety, which may prevent overeating.

Look at the calorie comparison of eight ounces of various types of milk as opposed to eight ounces of popular beverage options.

**Table 9.2 Calories in Eight Ounces of Various Beverages**

| Beverage, 8 ounces | Calories |
|---|---|
| Skim milk | 80 |
| 1 percent milk | 110 |
| Soy milk | 80 |
| Almond milk, unsweetened | 40 |
| Coconut milk | 90 |
| Hemp milk | 110 |
| Calcium-fortified orange juice | 110 |
| Soda, regular | 93 |
| Beverage, 8 ounces | Calories |
| Energy drink | 110 |
| Diet soda | 0 |
| Water | 0 |

An eight-ounce glass of skim milk has only eighty calories. Eight ounces of unsweetened, fortified almond milk has only forty calories. Both provide B vitamins, vitamin D, vitamin E, and potassium, along with over three hundred milligrams of calcium—a great nutritional investment for the meager calories. Of note, other than cow's milk and soy milk, milks like almond and coconut, provide minimal protein.

In contrast, eight ounces of regular soda provides ninety-three calories, all from high fructose corn syrup, with no nutritional value whatsoever. A one-ounce bag of potato chips contains one hundred fifty calories and minimal nutrition. A typical candy bar has two hundred calories. Instead of these high-fat, sugary, salty snacks or desserts, calcium-rich milk and a piece of fruit is a supernutritious replacement.

## CHILDREN AND PARENTS THINK DAIRY PRODUCTS ARE UNHEALTHY

Some people think that dairy products are full of pesticides and growth hormones. Many feel that dairy products cause allergies and digestive problems. There is no evidence yet to demonstrate that milk and dairy products contain unsafe levels of growth hormone used in dairy production.

Children may experience lactose intolerance, the inability to digest lactose—the sugar, or carbohydrate, in milk. Lactose intolerance is caused by the lack of lactase in the intestine. Lactase breaks down and helps digest lactose. Lactose intolerance can lead to bloating, cramps, and diarrhea—obviously, unpleasant occurrences on and off the tennis court.

Low-lactose and lactose-free milk are readily available for those who are lactose intolerant. Calcium-fortified soy, almond, hemp, coconut, and rice milk are also good options. The list goes on. Lactose content varies widely in dairy products. While fluid milk is higher in lactose, other dairy products like yogurt and cheese are much lower in lactose content and easier to digest. Lactase tablets and drops are also available. These tablets or drops are taken before eating dairy products to aid in lactose digestion.

## OTHER BEVERAGES ARE MORE APPEALING

Sparkling, colorful beverages have overtaken seemingly endless rows of grocery store shelving. Beverage companies target much of their marketing toward teens and young adults. Children and adults choose these sugary, artificially colored beverages over milk, juice, and water.

## VEGETARIAN KIDS

If children and teens follow vegan diets, calcium and vitamin D can come from nonanimal sources. These include calcium-fortified soy, almond, and rice milk; calcium-fortified juice; soy cheese, calcium-processed tofu, soy yogurt, and soy-based frozen desserts, to name a few. Ready-to-eat cereal, bread, and vegetables such as spinach, kale, and bok choy are also sources of calcium.

We know with certainty that milk contains more nutrition than just about any other beverage that exists. Those nutrients include protein, calcium, potassium, B vitamins, and phosphorous. Some even regard low-fat milk and yogurt as having superfood status.

Many parents and coaches incorporate a personal fitness trainer for their child's or teen's tennis training but neglect to include an RD or CSSD for nutritional counseling. Knowing the impact of sports nutrition on fitness level and athletic performance, coupled with the unique nutritional needs of children and teens, the support an RD or CSSD provides is invaluable. Their nutritional advice can teach healthy eating through the life span, giving children and teens the winning edge on and off the court.

The below websites for parents and children provide user-friendly nutrition advice, tips, and timely information.

1. www.Girlshealth.gov—health and nutrition tips specially for girls ages ten through sixteen by the US Department of Health and Human Services
2. www.KidsHealth.org—easy-to-understand, kid-focused information from health professionals
3. www.Nutrition.gov/youthweight—links to diet and weight management sites for children, teens, and adults
4. www.NourishInteractive.com (and in Spanish: www. NourishInteractive.com/languages/es)—fun games, blogs, and newsletters designed for children, with resources for parents and educators
5. www.EmpowerMe2b.org—offers a means for children to participate in polls and blogs and to share stories about the challenges and solutions to obesity; this site was created by the Alliance for a Healthier Generation
6. www.Bcm.edu/childrens-nutrition—the USDA has joined forces with Baylor College in Houston, Texas, to form the Children's Nutrition Research Center, one of

six in the country; this site provides a free subscription to *Nutrition and Your Child*, an online newsletter with informative nutrition articles geared to parents and children

Gabriel, who was introduced in the beginning of the chapter, is a prime candidate for sports nutrition counseling. He surely needs guidance on how to safely gain weight, working with his short list of food preferences to adapt a high-energy eating plan individualized to his needs. He must learn how the timing of foods and fluids affects his on-court energy level, stamina, and mental focus.

Children and teens are impressionable. Once they experience the benefits of sports nutrition, especially with positive tennis results, these rewards will reinforce favorable eating habits over the life span.

# 10

## Nutrient Timing for Optimal Tennis Performance

**It's not who you are that holds you back,
it's who you think you're not.**
—Unknown

Brittney is a seventeen-year-old tennis player who has had tremendous success as a court-one singles player for her high school team. She competed in countless tournaments as a star junior player—so many that she and her family have a difficult time remembering all her special victorious moments. There is one, however, that is indelibly imprinted in their memories. Brittney was scheduled to play two matches at a prestigious national invitational tournament, one in the morning and one in the afternoon. Unforeseen circumstances occurred, as they often do in tournament play, including an hour rain delay in the morning. Her marathon three-set match that lasted over two and a half hours compounded the delay even further. Having only a pastry and coffee early in the morning, Brittney came off the court starving and feeling light-headed. Yet she only had an hour before her next match. Her family rushed her off to a popular Mexican restaurant where Brittney scarfed down two burritos, tortilla chips with queso and salsa, and a large, fizzy soda. Brittney was more ready for a nap than another tennis match. As she proceeded to play her next match, she started belching, passing gas, and feeling nauseated. Each time she ran or jolted, her stomach felt the same undulation. During the match, Brittney repeatedly went to the bathroom. Feeling so sick to her stomach, she had to forfeit her second match and the potential for a prestigious title.

Nutrition for tennis performance is only as effective as what is practiced on and off the court. This chapter translates the timing of food and nutrients before, during, and after tennis play into winning sample menus and meal plans. Nutrient timing is well known in sports nutrition. Research has demonstrated that timed ingestion of nutrients, including carbohydrates and protein, significantly affects our bodies' adaptive response to exercise.[222] Sports nutrition works. Utilize food and fluids to enhance your tennis performance.

Nutrient timing requires methodical planning and discipline. If you need help, seek assistance from an RD or CSSD to customize meal timing and menus to meet your individual need for calories, food preferences, weight target, and supplementation. You may have specific practices (such as vegetarian, vegan, kosher, gluten-free), food allergies, medical/surgical history, and/or disease-specific conditions—such as asthma, celiac disease, or diabetes, kidney, or heart disease—requiring dietary modification. The following tennis scenarios we all face describe how to practice nutrient timing and why it can make or break your match play.

## TWO DAYS PREMATCH/PRETOURNAMENT

Most often, a tennis draw is known only a day or two before match play. Players who want the winning edge need to plan their competitive tennis nutrition at least two days ahead of event day. Always remember, being sports nutrition tennis ready starts several days prior to game day. Nutrition neglect cannot be compensated for a few minutes before a match.

## Goals

- *Fuel up.* Increase carbohydrate intake for glycogen synthesis and storage in the liver and muscle. Studies show that exercise intensity, pace, and work output decrease as glycogen levels diminish. Consume high-carbohydrate meals one to three days prior to event to maximize glycogen storage. Preevent meals should provide 8–10 grams per kilogram of body weight per day.[223] As an example, if you weigh seventy kilograms, you would need a preexercise diet containing 560–700 grams of carbohydrate. To put this in perspective, one slice of bread or a half cup of cooked pasta has about 15–20 grams of carbohydrate.
- *Protein.* Obtain essential amino acids from vegetable or lean animal protein sources, such as fish, chicken breast, lean beef, and pork. Vegetable protein sources include beans, soy, and grains like quinoa. However, if the high fiber content of beans and legumes makes them difficult to digest, resort to more easily digestible sources. Consuming both carbohydrate and protein prior to exercise has been shown to produce greater levels of muscle protein synthesis.[224]
- *Good hydration.* Drink extra fluids for good hydration well before a match. Fluids with nutrition are good choices and include 100 percent juice, milk, coconut water, and, of course, water. Start doing the urine color check now.
- *Balance rest with practice.* This will ensure that muscles are replenished with glycogen while the body rests and recovers for game day.

***Sample Menus.*** Below are nutrient-rich supercharged menus with the proper composition of carbohydrates, protein, fat, vitamins, minerals, and phytonutrients for pretennis nutrition.

## 2,500 Calorie Sample Menus for Tennis Players

| Day 1 Breakfast: | Day 2 Breakfast: |
|---|---|
| 1 whole-grain bagel*<br>2 tablespoons natural peanut<br>peanut butter<br>1/2 grapefruit<br>1 cup of coffee, decaf, or tea<br>(optional) | 1 cup oatmeal<br>1 tablespoon each dried<br>cranberries, walnuts, and<br>crushed flaxseed<br>8 ounces yogurt<br>1/2 cup fortified orange juice |
| **Day 1 Lunch:** | **Day 2 Lunch:** |
| 1 1/2 cups mixed salad greens:<br>spring mix with kale<br>fresh vegetables of choice:<br>tomato, shredded carrot, beets<br>4 ounces sliced grilled chicken<br>2 tablespoons balsamic vinegar/<br>olive oil dressing<br>15 whole-wheat crackers*<br>1 cup skim, soy, rice, or almond<br>milk<br>**Snack:** 4 tablespoon hummus<br>with 2 oz. pretzels | 2 slices whole-grain bread*<br>3 ounces turkey, 1 tablespoon<br>mayo<br>1 oz. sweet-potato chips<br>apple slices (1 medium apple)<br>**Snack:** 2 oatmeal-raisin cookies*<br>1 cup skim, soy, rice, or almond<br>milk |
| **Day 1 Dinner:** | **Day 2 Dinner:** |
| 1 1/2 cups cooked pasta* with<br>2/3 cup Bolognese sauce<br>1/2 cup steamed broccoli<br>1 cup frozen yogurt | 4 ounces cooked salmon w/fresh<br>herbs and lemon<br>1 large baked sweet potato<br>1 tablespoon brown sugar,<br>1 teaspoon butter<br>1/2 cup green peas<br>3/4 cup ice cream |
| **Evening Snack:** | **Evening Snack:** |
| 2/3 bowl whole-grain cereal*<br>(e.g., toasted oats, bran flakes,<br>granola)<br>1 cup skim, soy, rice, or almond<br>milk and 1 banana | 1 yogurt smoothie<br>20 whole-grain snack chips |

*These foods can easily be replaced with gluten-free bread or cereal for those with gluten sensitivity. Those with lactose intolerance or who follow a dairy-free diet can get calcium and vitamin D from fortified orange juice, soy, almond, hemp, or rice milk.

## GAME DAY

Your nutrition regimen can vary depending on what time your tennis match is played. Examples of common tennis match scenarios are listed below. Tennis nutrition timing tips accompany each case. Key goals include maintaining blood glucose and muscle glycogen stores during exercise, both of which are major determinants of athletic performance. With a modest amount of planning, nutrient timing can give you the performance edge.

### SCENARIO 1: TENNIS MATCH AT 8:30 A.M.

Goals:
- **Fuel up.** Eat adequate carbohydrates the night before and morning of your match. Utilize the sample dinner menus for ideas. Eat a healthy, balanced dinner meal with lean or vegetable protein, complex carbohydrates, and unsaturated fats.

  On the morning of, prevent feeling heavy, bloated, or sluggish by eating a light, easy-to-digest breakfast at least an hour before your morning match. This gives you time for your body to focus its energy on digestion before tennis. Save the heavy bacon-and-eggs breakfast for a nonmatch day. Eating breakfast does the following:
  a.  It restores liver glycogen in the morning when liver glycogen is depleted from an overnight fast from a good night's sleep.

b. Along with replenishing glycogen reserves from the night before, breakfast increases glycogen stores needed for impending exercise.

c. It prevents hunger and low blood sugar.

d. It gives you a physiological boost of energy.

If you are not an early breakfast eater, try a smoothie with fruit and yogurt thirty minutes prior to your match. If that is not tolerated, ensure a healthy, complete dinner the night before and have thirty grams of easily digestible, carbohydrate-rich food before your match, such as a large banana or two pieces of toast. Pack several bottles of sports drink. Bring healthy snacks in your tennis bag, such as a banana, granola bar, dried fruit, and/or a bag of pretzels. Use these snacks when you start having an appetite both before and during play. Eat a snack before hunger pangs set in.

Athletes who have reactive hypoglycemia should adapt their carbohydrate-rich foods accordingly. If you experience hypoglycemia by eating so many carbohydrates, choose low-glycemic, easily digestible carbohydrate foods an hour before exercise. (Page 148 gives examples of low glycemic foods.)

- **Good hydration.** Drink enough fluids the night before and morning of the match. Continue to do the urine color check. Also, check the weather report far ahead of match day. Sunny, hot, humid weather results in much greater sweat loss compared to a cloudy, cooler forecast. Hydrate accordingly.

## SCENARIO 2: TENNIS MATCH AT NOON

### Goals:
- **Fuel up.** Eat a good breakfast in the morning, several hours before your noon match. Cereal, fruit, and milk; fruit, toast, and a scrambled egg; yogurt and fresh fruit are simple breakfasts that provide good nutrition in an easily digestible meal. Again, even with a later match, save the large traditional bacon-and-eggs breakfast for a nonmatch morning. Try the helpful preexercise prescription for carbohydrates by eating one to four grams of carbohydrate per kilogram of body weight one to four hours before exercise:

> 1 g carb/kg body weight—one hour before exercise
> 2 g carb/kg body weight—two hours before exercise
> 3 g carb/kg body weight—three hours before exercise
> 4 g carb/kg body weight—four hours before exercise[225]

A noon match means tennis is played during traditional lunch hours. Plan ahead. One to two hours before the match, have a light meal, similar to the nutrition in the breakfast outlined above, with carbohydrates, protein, and a small amount of fat. A half or whole sandwich with lean protein or a smoothie with yogurt will stave off hunger while supplying fuel and nutrients.

Plan your midmorning, prematch nutrition around the timing of your first meal. For example, if you are an early riser and eat breakfast at six thirty, you have plenty of time to eat and digest a light lunch meal an hour or two before the match. In contrast, if you tend to sleep late and have a good breakfast at ten o'clock, then a second meal can be replaced by a carbohydrate-rich snack, such as a banana, apple, pretzels, or rice cakes. Always have healthy snacks in your tennis bag. This will give you the reassurance that you will have instant fuel a few steps away.

- **Good hydration.** Drink enough fluids during the day to maintain hydration prior to match. Since the heat index is highest between 10:00 a.m. and 2:00 p.m., be prepared to hydrate more before, during, and after a noon match.

## SCENARIO 3: TENNIS MATCH AT 4:00 P.M.

### Goals:
- **Fuel up.** Not surprisingly, stay on your meal plan by eating a good breakfast and lunch. One to two hours prior to a 4:00 p.m. match, have a light meal or snack with carbohydrate. Because this could be a second or even a third match on a tournament day, finding time to eat and drink between matches can be at a premium. When there are fewer than eight hours between matches, you should consume carbohydrates immediately after the first match to optimize recovery.[226]

  Between checking scores, catching up with friends, and resting, nutrition can fall low on the list of priorities. Consume the recovery snacks or minimeals outlined on page 132 for ideas.

- **Good hydration.** Drink plenty of fluids between matches, including water and sports drinks. Continue to do the urine color check throughout the day. If this is the second or third match, be sure to catch up on your hydration by drinking plenty of fluids between matches.

  Be sure to include enough sodium and potassium in your meals or fluids to replenish electrolyte losses in sweat. Muscle cramping is the result of sodium and potassium loss, which is more pronounced toward the end of tournament day when fluids and electrolytes have not been sufficiently replenished.

• **Make every attempt to cool off indoors.** In the tournament environment, this can be challenging. Options include an air-conditioned restaurant, pro shop, car, lounge, or locker room. This helps evaporate sweat, which cools the body, and prevents further sweat loss. (Refer to chapter 7 for the type and amount of fluids to drink during all-day tennis.)

## DURING MATCH PLAY

Studies show that as exercise increases beyond sixty minutes, outside carbohydrate sources become important in maintaining blood glucose levels and muscle glycogen stores.[227] Carbohydrates during rigorous tennis play should supply thirty to sixty grams per hour. This dose can easily be achieved by drinking eight to sixteen ounces of a sports drink every fifteen minutes of exercise or the equivalent of the carbohydrate-containing snacks listed in chapter 8.[228]

Further, research suggests that ingesting different types of carbohydrates during exercise enhances exercise performance, particularly in endurance exercise. Experts believe a combination of different types of carbohydrates may also improve performance in stop-and-go sports like tennis that require repeated bouts of high-intensity, short-duration effort.[229] Serving a ball, running to the net to punch a volley, and engaging in a twenty-shot rally are examples of this type of effort.

Combining carbohydrates is much simpler than it sounds. A popular sports drink contains a combination of carbohydrates, including maltodextrin, sucrose, and glucose. This combination of carbohydrates may be more effective than having food or drink with a single type of carbohydrate. Have a variety of food and fluid sources of carbohydrates in your tennis bag, such as sports drinks, sports beans and gels, bananas, pretzels, and granola bars.

## POST-TENNIS

Whether you are victorious after a hard-fought tennis match or not, post-tennis nutrition remains a necessity for several reasons. Good nutrition efficiently replenishes fluids, energy, carbohydrates, protein, and electrolytes lost during physical activity. During this window of anabolic opportunity, post-tennis carbohydrates and protein in the form of amino acids aid in fast muscle synthesis, repair, and recovery. This is because of the following:

a. Blood flow to muscles is much greater after exercise.
b. Muscle cells are more likely to take up glucose made from the foods we eat.
c. Muscles are more sensitive to the effects of insulin, which promotes glycogen synthesis.[230]

A good meal after tennis also satiates a hearty appetite worked up from hours of hard work on the court. Postexercise nutrition is especially important if subsequent matches are played that day or the following day.

**Goals:**
- **Replenish carbohydrates.** Postexercise consumption of carbohydrates replenishes fuel needed to engage in the rest of the day's activities or carry you through another match later in the day. Refueling for peak tournament play is essential.
- **Repair and recover worn muscles with protein intake.** Intake of essential amino acids from protein has been shown to stimulate robust increases in muscle protein synthesis.

Protein combined with postexercise carbohydrate has also been shown to assist in muscle glycogen synthesis to a greater extent than carbohydrates alone.[231]

- **Hydrate** for fluid repletion. Bergeron suggests hydrating 1.5 times your postexercise hydration needs. (Chapter 7 provides guidelines for hydration needs postexercise.)
- **Satisfy your appetite!** Enjoy your favorite healthy meal after a hard-earned tennis victory.

Brittney, introduced at the beginning of the chapter, learned her nutrient timing lesson the hard way after she had to forfeit her tournament match due to gastrointestinal distress. She now knows to plan ahead days before her event; eat a healthy breakfast with carbohydrates and small amounts of protein and fat on match morning; pack nutritious, high-carbohydrate snacks in her tennis bag; and not choose spicy, gassy, high-fat foods for lunch right before her match—no matter how hungry she is.

# 11

## WINNING TENNIS NUTRITION FOR LIFE

**I guess I was probably the first woman to lift weights and do circuit training and to run the sand hills.**
—Margaret Court

Jean is sixty-nine years old and lives to play tennis. The blistering Florida heat will not keep this feisty senior away from the tennis court. A retired schoolteacher, Jean has exhibited that same classroom discipline in so many of her health behaviors. She does not drink alcohol or smoke and rarely eats junk food. She keeps her weight at a steady ideal set point, although she admits finding it more challenging in her senior years. She judiciously drills at her tennis club, playing at every opportunity she finds. She still competes in singles at an elite level in local leagues and state competition, beating players less than half her age with her mental toughness, skill, and craftiness. Jean has never had a tennis injury—not even tennis elbow. She is a perfect example of how nutrition, fitness, and discipline have paid tremendous dividends in her being a happily active and competitive tennis player in her golden years.

A fitting closure, exemplifying how fitness and nutrition influence tennis performance over a lifetime, is the case of sixty-nine-year-old Jean. However, even Jean's story cannot top that of inspiring eighty-six-year-old Doris "Jane" Lutz. Jane Lutz is currently (as of April 2015) the International Tennis Foundation's (ITF) number-one female player in the women's eighty-five-year-old singles category. Jane recently won both the prestigious ITF world individual singles and doubles titles in 2012. She is the captain of USTA's Doris Hart team, which travels all over the world to compete in international seniors play. Lutz has recently represented the United States in international play in Turkey, Croatia, and Austria. Jane has won sixty-five gold balls in her career—each gold ball represents a national title. She also has bragging rights to twenty-five silver balls and twenty-four bronze balls—second- and third-place trophies, respectively.

This peppy tennis dynamo only started playing at the age of fifty-five—an age when many adults start slowing their tennis game down. Instead, recognizing her talent, Jane pursued tennis with foremost dedication. Jane had a late tennis start for a reason. She raised four children during her extremely happy sixty-year marriage with former baseball pro and Cleveland Indians coach, the late Joe Lutz. In addition to raising her four children, a more than full-time job itself, Jane also retired as a schoolteacher before starting her tennis career.

I interviewed Jane at our tennis club in Sarasota, Florida.[232] Florida is a mecca for tennis greats, young and old. I asked Jane the inevitable burning question: what's your secret? How does someone who picks up a racquet at the age of fifty-five become a world champion at the age of eighty-five? Looking as if she would disappoint me in her much-anticipated response, Jane said, "I have no secrets." There have been no notable supplements, diet regimens, or exercise fads she has ever considered trying. In contrast, her tennis fortitude is the result of her lifelong commitment to exercise, good nutrition, and positive attitude.

Jane's responses exemplify the foundation from which great tennis comes. Her lifestyle has been characterized by the following:

- No smoking and no alcohol.
- Eating regular, balanced meals. Never skipping meals or trying a fad diet, ever.
- Eating what she likes in the proper portions without worrying about it. This includes having two to three cans of cola per day, her only self-regarded dietary vice. Jane more than makes up for this "bad habit she cannot shake" with the positive aspects of the rest of her diet and training regimen.
- Exercise. Her rigorous training routine includes hitting and tennis drills two to three hours per day, frequently capped off with an hour of serving practice.
- Staying within her physical limits. Jane trusts what her body can physically manage and listens to its signals for rest and recovery. Jane has been injury-free in her thirty years of playing competitive tennis.
- Having a positive attitude. Admittedly, Jane says her life has been a very happy one, which has influenced her attitude about the game, on and off the court. Her demeanor exudes a calm confidence and mental grit, which has helped her succeed on and off the tennis court.
- Loving tennis. Jane believes her success has come because she plays tennis for the pure reason that she loves to play. She does not compete for anyone else except herself. She does not play to impress anyone. She recognizes that, at all age levels, many compete for other reasons besides the sheer enjoyment of playing. She vows that she will continue to play tennis until the day she stops loving the game.

Although many of us will not come near having the tennis fortune bestowed upon Jane, her story inspires tennis players of all ages. Through having a commonsense yet disciplined approach to eating and fitness, she has reaped rewards beyond anyone's dreams for tennis success—and longevity.

# Selected Bibliography

Academy of Nutrition and Dietetics. "Fad Diet Timeline." Accessed January 25, 2015. http://www.eatright.org/nnm/ games /timeline/index.html.

Academy of Nutrition and Dietetics Sports, Cardiovascular, and Nutrition Practice Group. "The Female Athlete Triad." January 2010. Accessed February 15, 2015. http://www. scandpg.org/sports-nutrition/sports-nutrition-fact-sheets/.

Academy of Nutrition and Dietetics Sports, Cardiovascular and Nutrition Practice Group. "The Sunny Side of Vitamin D." January 2011. Accessed February 15, 2015. http://www. scandpg.org/sports-nutrition/sports-nutrition-fact-sheets/.

Academy of Nutrition and Dietetics Sports, Cardiovascular, and Nutrition Practice Group. "Sport Foods." 2015. Accessed February 15, 2015. http://www. scandpg.org/sports-nutrition/ sports-nutrition-fact-sheets/.

Academy of Nutrition and Dietetics. "Position of the Academy of Nutrition and Dietetics: Dietary Fatty Acids for Healthy Adults." *Journal of the Academy of Nutrition and Dietetics* 114, no. 1 (2014): 136–153. doi:10.1016/j.jand.2013.11.001.

Academy of Nutrition and Dietetics. "Position of the Academy of Nutrition and Dietetics: Use of Nutritive and Non-Nutritive Sweeteners." *Journal of the Academy of Nutrition and Dietetics* 112, no. 5 (2012): 739–758.

Albers, Michelle. "Food Cravings, Habits and Emotions." Institute of Natural Resources. http://www.INRseminars. com (seminar, Bradenton, Florida, March 2014).

Albers, Susan. Accessed November 18, 2014. htttp://www. eatingmindfully.com/mindfuleatingplate.

American Academy of Pediatrics. Press Release. "American Academy of Pediatrics Weighs in for the First Time on Organic Foods for Children." October 22, 2012. http://www. aap.org/en-us/about-the-aap/aap-press-room.

American Bottled Water Association. Press Release. "Bottled Water Sales and Consumption Projected to Increase in 2014, Expected to be the Number One Packaged Drink by 2016." December 4, 2014. Accessed May 13, 2015. http://www. bottledwater.org/bottled-water-sales-and-consumption-projected-increase-2014-expected-to-be-number-one-packaged-drink.

American Chemical Society. "Coconut Water is an Excellent Sports Drink—For Light Exercise." *Science Daily*. August 20, 2012. http://www.sciencedaily.com/releases/2012/08 /120820143902.htm.

American College of Sports Medicine. "Position Stand: Nutrition and Athletic Performance." *Medicine and Science in Sports and Exercise* 41, no. 3 (2009): 709–731.

American College of Sports Medicine. "American College of Sports Medicine Position Stand on Exercise and Fluid Replacement." *Medicine and Science in Sports and Exercise* 38, no. 2 (2007): 377–390. doi:108:249.208.148.

American College of Sports Medicine Consumer Information Committee. "Selecting and Effectively Using Sports Drinks, Carbohydrate Gels and Energy Bars." 2011. Accessed February 21, 2015. http://www.acsm.org/docs/brochures/ ... using-sports ... gels-and-energy-bars.pdf.

American College of Sports Medicine/National Athletic Association. "Current Comment: Eating Disorders."

Accessed January 25, 2015. http://www.acsm.org/docs/ current-comments /eatingdisorders.pdf.

American Diabetes Association. "Glycemic Index and Diabetes." Last modified March 14, 2014. http://www.diabetes.org/ glycemic-index-and-diabetes.html.

American Heart Association. "Know Your Fats." October 11, 2012. http://www.heart.org/HEARTORG/conditions/cholesterol/ PreventionTreatmentofHighCholesterol/Know-Your-Fats/.

American Heart Association. "What Your Cholesterol Levels Mean." October 11, 2012. http://www.heart.org/ HEARTORG/conditions/cholesterol /aboutcholesterol/ What-Your-Cholesterol-Levels-Mean/.

American Medical Association. Press Release. "American Medical Association Affirms High Fructose Corn Syrup Not a Unique Contributor to Obesity." June 18, 2008.

American Psychiatric Association. *Diagnostic and Statistical Manual of Mental Disorders*, 5th ed., 2013.

Amidor, Toby. "Clean Eating." *Today's Dietitian* 15, no. 5 (2013): 10–11.

Aragon, Alan A., and Brad Jon Schoenfeld. "Nutrient Timing Revisited: Is There a Postexercise Anabolic Window?" *Journal of the International Society of Sports Nutrition* 10, no. 5 (2013): 1–11.

Arias, Jimmy. Interview by Grace Lee. 2014.

Bailey, R. L., K. W. Dodd, J. A. Goldman, J. J. Gahche, J. T. Dwyer, A. J. Moshfegh, C. T. Sempos, and M. F. Picciano. "Estimation of Total Usual Calcium and Vitamin D Intakes in the United States." *Journal of Nutrition* 140, no. 4 (2010): 817–822.

Baranski, M., D. Tober-Srednicka, N. Volakakis, C. Seal, R. Sanderson, G. B. Stewart, C. Benbrook, et al. "Higher Antioxidant and Lower Cadmium Concentrations and Lower Incidence of Pesticide Residues in Organically Grown Crops."

*British Journal of Nutrition* 125, no. 5 (2014): 794–811. doi: 10.1017/S00007114514001366.Epub 2014 Jun 26.

Bar-Or, Oded. "Nutrition for Children and Adolescent Athletes." Sports Science Exchange #77 (2000). Gatorade Sport Science Institute. Accessed January 15, 2014. http://www.gssiweb.org.

Bergeron, Michael. "Heat and Hydration in Young Tennis Players." American College of Sports Medicine Current Comment. Accessed January 28, 2015. http://www.acsm.org/docs/current-comments /heatandhydration.pdf.

Bergeron, Michael. United States Tennis Association. "Playing Tennis in the Heat: How to Manage Water and Electrolyte Losses." Accessed January 28, 2015. http://www.usta.com/Improve-Your-Game/Sport-Science/114718_Nutrition_Playing_Tennis_In_The_Heat_How_To_Manage_Water_and_Electrolyte_Losses/.

Bollettieri, Nick. Interview by Grace Lee. 2012 and January 23, 2015.

Burke, Louise M., John A. Hawley, Stephen H. Wong, and Asker E. Jeukendrup. "Carbohydrates for Training and Competition." *Journal of Sports Science* 29, Suppl 1 (2011): S17–27. doi: 10.1080/02640414.2011.585473.Epub 2011 Jun 9.

Campbell, B. "International Society of Sports Nutrition Position Stand: Energy Drinks." *Journal of the Society of International Sports Nutrition* 10, no. 1 (2013). doi: 10.1186/1550-2783-10-1.

Campbell, Bill, Richard B. Kreider, Tim Ziegenfuss, Paul LaBounty, Mike Roberts, Darren Burke, Jamie Landis, Hector Lopez, and Jose Antonio. "International Society of Sports Nutrition Position Stand: Protein and Exercise." *Journal of the International Society of Sports Nutrition* 4, no. 8 (2007). doi:10.1186/1550-2783-4-8.

Center for Disease Control and Prevention. "Adult Obesity Facts." Last reviewed August 13, 2013. http://www.cdc.gov/obesity /date/adult.html.

Center for Disease Control and Prevention. "State Indicator Report on Fruits and Vegetables." 2009. Accessed January 15, 2015. http://www.cdc.gov/nutrition/downloads/State IndicatorReport2009.pdf.

Center for Disease Control and Prevention. "Fact Sheets— Alcohol Use and Public Health." Last reviewed November 7, 2014. http://www.cdc.gov/alcohol /fact-sheets/.

Center for Disease Control and Prevention. "Assessing Your Weight." Last reviewed October 21, 2014. http://www.cdc. gov/healthyweight/assessing /index.html.

Center for Disease Control and Prevention. "Childhood Obesity Facts." Last reviewed December 11, 2014. http://www.cdc. gov/healthyyouth/obesity/ fact.htm.

Center for Science in the Public Interest. "Caffeine Content of Food and Drugs." Accessed January 25, 2015. http://www. cspinet.org/new/cafchart.htm.

Center for Science in the Public Interest. "FDA Urged to Determine Safe Limits on High Fructose Corn Syrup." 2013. http://www.cspinet.org/new /201302131.html.

Chella, David, and Joseph Murray. "Celiac Disease on the Rise." Mayo Clinic: Discovery's Edge. July 2010.

Chowdury, Rajiv, Samantha Warnakula, Setor Kunutsor, Fransesca Crowe, Heather A. Ward, Laura Johnson, Oscar H. Franco, et al. "Association of Dietary, Circulating and Supplement Fatty Acids with Coronary Artery Risk: A Systemic Review and Meta-Analysis." *Annals of Internal Medicine* 160, no. 6 (2014): 398–406. doi:10.7326/M13-1788.

Clark, Kristine. "Sports Nutrition: The Power to Influence Exercise Performance." Conagra webinar. May 21, 2014. http://www.conagrafoodscienceinstitute.com.

Clark, Nancy. *Sports Nutrition Guidebook*. 5th ed. Champaign, IL: Human Kinetics, 2014.

Cloutier, Marissa, and Eve Adamson. *The Mediterranean Diet*. New York: Harper, 2004.

Cook, Eliza, and Rachel Dunifon. "Do Family Meals Really Make a Difference?" *Parenting in Context*. Cornell University Cooperative Extension. 2012.

Craig, W. J., and A. R. Mangels. "Position on the Academy of Nutrition and Dietetics: Vegetarian Diets." *Journal of the Academy of Nutrition and Dietetics* 109, no. 7 (2009): 1266–1282.

Davis, Bob. Interview by Grace Lee. June 2013.

Davis, Tiffany Dabek. Interview by Grace Lee. October 2014.

DeMarco, Helen. "American College of Sports Medicine Current Comment: Pre-Event Meals." Accessed January 28, 2015. http://www.acsm.org/docs/currentcomments/ preeventmeals.pdf.

Denke, Margo A. "Metabolic Effects of High-Protein, Low Carbohydrate Diets." *The American Journal of Cardiology* 88 (2001): 59–61.

Djokovic, Novak. *Serve to Win: The 14-Day Gluten-Free Plan for Physical and Mental Excellence*. New York: Zinc Ink, 2013.

Ejinde, B. Op't, L. Vergawen, and P. Hespel. "Creatine Loading Does Not Impact on Stroke Performance in Tennis." *International Journal of Sports Medicine* 22, no. 1 (2001): 76–80.

Environmental Working Group Executive Summary. "EWG's 2014 Shopper's Guide to Pesticides in Produce." Reviewed April 2014. Accessed January 12, 2015. http://www.ewg.org /foodnews /summary.php.

Estruch, Ramon, Emilio Ros, Jodi Salas-Salvado, Maria-Isabel Covas, Dolores Corella, Fernando Aros, Enrique Gomez-Gracia, et al. "Primary Prevention of Cardiovascular Disease with a Mediterranean Diet." *New England Journal of Medicine* 368, no. 14 (2013): 1279–1290. doi: 10.1056 / NEJMoa1200303.

Farrow, Damian. "Caffeine, Carbohydrate and Cooling Use During Prolonged Simulated Tennis." *International Journal of Sports Physiology and Performance* 2, no. 4 (2008): 423–438.

Food and Agricultural Organization/World Health Organization. "Fruits and Vegetables for Health." Report of a Joint FAO/WHO Workshop, September 1–3, 2004. Accessed February 4, 2015. http://www. who.int/dietphysicalactivity/publications/fruit_vegetables_report.pdf.

Food and Agricultural Organization of the United Nations. "International Year of Quinoa, 2013." Accessed February 8, 2015. http://www.fao.org/quinoa-2013/en/.

Food and Agricultural Organization Newsroom. "Livestock, A Major Threat to the Environment." Accessed February 15, 2015. http://www. fao.org/newsroom/en/news/2006/1000448/index.html.

Food and Drug Administration. "Tips for Dietary Supplement Users." Last updated April 23, 2014. http://www.fda.gov/Food/DietarySupplements/ UsingDietarySupplements/ucm110567.htm.

Food and Drug Administration. "Using the Nutrition Facts Food Label." Accessed January 25, 2015. http://www.fda. gov/downloads /Food/ResourcesForYou /Consumers/ UCM275396.pdf.

Food and Drug Administration. "FDA Targets Trans Fat in Processed Foods." November 7, 2013. http://www.fda.gov/ForConsumers /ConsumerUpdates/ucm372915.htm.

Food and Drug Administration. "Talking About Trans Fat: What You Need to Know." Last updated December 18, 2014. http://www.fda.gov/Food/IngredientsPackagingLabeling/LabelingNutrition/ucm079609.htm.

Food and Drug Administration. "Proposed Changes to the Nutrition Facts Label." Last updated August 1, 2014. http://www.fda.gov /Food/GuidanceRegulation/GuidanceDocumentsRegulatoryInformation/Labeling Nutrition/ucm385663.htm.

Franz, Mary. "Nutrition, Inflammation and Disease." *Today's Dietitian* 16, no. 2 (2014): 44.

Fuhrman, Joel, and Deana M. Ferreri. "Fueling the Vegetarian (Vegan) Athlete." *Current Sports Medicine Reports (American College of Sports Medicine)* 9, no. 4 (2010): 233–241.

Getz, Lindsey. "Deciphering Whole Grain Food Labels—Separating Fact from Fiction." *Today's Dietitian* 14, no. 6 (2012): 44.

Goldstein, Erica R., Tim Ziegenfuss, Doug Kalman, Richard Kreider, Bill Campbell, Colin Wilborn, Lem Taylor, et al. "International Society of Sports Nutrition Position Stand: Caffeine and Performance." *Journal of the International Society of Sports Nutrition* 7, no. 5 (2010).

Graham, Terry, and Lawrence Spriet. "Caffeine and Exercise." Sports Science Exchange #60. Gatorade Sport Science Institute. http://www.gssiweb.org.

Gunders, Dana. "Wasted: How America is Losing Up to 40 Percent of Its Food from Farm to Fork to Landfill." Natural Resources Defense Council (NRDC), Issue Paper, August 2012. IP:12-06-B. http://www.nrdc.org/food/files/wasted-food-ip.pdf.

Hammond, Alan L. "How Does Caffeine Affect Your Tennis Game?" May 2, 2008. US Professional Tennis Association (USPTA). http://www.tennis-health.com/Articles/tabid/128/Articles/HowDoesCaffeineAffectYourTennisGame.htm.

Hammons, Amber J., and Barbara H. Fiese. "Is Frequency of Shared Family Meals Related to the Nutritional Health of Children and Adolescents?" *Pediatrics* 127, no. 6 (2011): e1565–e1574. doi: 10.1542/peds2010-1440.

Harvard University School of Public Health. "Health Gains from Whole Grains." Accessed February 8, 2015. http://www.hsph.harvard.edu/nutritionsource/health-gains-from-whole-grains/.

Harvard University School of Public Health. "Harvard Healthy Eating Plate." Accessed February 5, 2015. http://www.health.harvard.edu/plate/health-hearing-plate.

Harvard University School of Public Health. "Vegetables and Fruits: Get Plenty Every Day." Accessed March 8, 2015. http://www.hsph.harvard.edu/nutritionsource /vegetables-full story.

Hoffman, Jay R., and Michael J. Flavo. "Protein—Which Is Best?" International Society of Sports Nutrition Symposium, June 2005. *Journal of Sports Science and Medicine* 3 (2004): 118–130.

Holick, Michael F. "Resurrection of Vitamin D Deficiency and Rickets." *Journal of Clinical Investigation* 116, no. 8 (2006): 2062–2072.

Holyand, Alexa, Louise Dye, and Clare L. Lawton. "A Systemic Review of the Effect of Breakfast on the Cognitive Performance of Children and Adolescents." *Nutrition Research Reviews* 22 (2009): 220–243. doi: 10.1017/S0954422409990175.

Hornery, D. J., D. Farrow, I. Mujika, and W. Young. "Fatigue in Tennis: Mechanism of Fatigue and Effects on Performance." *Sports Medicine* 7 (2007): 199–212.

Ichinose-Kuwahara, Tomoko, Yoshimitsu Inoue, Yoshiko Iseki, Sachi Hara, Yukio Ogura, and Narihiko Kondo. "Sex Differences on the Effects of Physical Training on Sweat Gland Responses During a Graded Exercise." *Experimental Physiology* 19, no. 10 (2010): 1026-1032. doi: 10:1113/ expphysiol.2010.053710.

Institute of Medicine. "Dietary Reference Intakes: Vitamins." Last updated October 12, 2014. http://www.iom.edu/-/ media/Files/Activity%20Files/Nutrition/DRIs/DRI.

Institute of Medicine. "Dietary Reference Intakes for Calcium and Vitamin D Report Brief." Posted November 30, 2010. http:// www.iom.edu/Reports/2010/Dietary-Reference-Intakes-for-Calcium-and-Vitamin-D.aspx.

International Tennis Foundation. "Anti-Doping Programme." Accessed February 8, 2015. http://www.itftennis.com/ antidoping.

International Tennis Foundation. "Nutrition." Accessed January 28, 2015. http://www.itftennis.com/scienceandmedicine/nutrition/.

Jeukendrup, Asker. "Multiple Transportable Carbohydrates and Their Benefits—Sports Science Exchange #108." Gatorade Sports Science Institute. Accessed January 25, 2015. http://www.gssiweb.org/sports-science-exchange.

Kalman, Douglas S., Samantha Feldman, Diane R. Krieger, and Richard J. Bloomer. "Comparison of Coconut Water and a Carbohydrate-Electrolyte Sport Drink on Measures of Hydration and Physical Performance on Exercise-Trained Men." *Journal of the International Society of Sports Nutrition* 9, no. 1 (2012): 1–10. doi: 10.1186/1550-27839-9-1.

Kerksick, Chad, Travis Harvey, Jeff Stout, Bill Campbell, Colin Wilborn, Richard Kreider, Doug Kalman, Tim Ziegenfuss, and Hector Lopez. "International Society of Sports Nutrition Position Stand: Nutrient Timing." *Journal of the International Society of Sports Nutrition* 5, no. 17 (2008). doi:10.1186/1550-2783-5-17.

Killip, Shersten, John Bennett, and Mara Chambers. "Iron Deficiency Anemia." *American Family Physician* 75, no. 5 (2007): 671–678.

Kleiner, Susan. "The Role of Red Meat in the Athlete's Diet." Gatorade Sports Science Institute Sports Science Exchange #58, no. 5 (1995). http://www.gssiweb.org/en/sports-science-exchange.

Kovacs, Mark S. "A Review of Fluid and Hydration in Competitive Tennis." *International Journal of Sports Physiology and Performance* 3 (2008): 413–423.

Kovacs, Mark S. "Applied Physiology of Tennis Performance." *British Journal of Sports Medicine* 40 (2006b): 381–385.

Kovacs, Mark S. "Carbohydrate Intake and Tennis: Are There Benefits?" *British Journal of Sports Medicine* 40, no. 5 (2006): e13. doi:10.1136 /bjsm.2005.023921.

Kovacs, Mark S. "Hydration and Temperature in Tennis—A Practical Review." *Journal of Sports Science and Medicine* 5, no. 1 (2006): 1–9.

Kovacs, Mark S., and Lindsay A. Baker. "Recovery Interventions and Strategies for Improved Tennis Performance." *British Journal of Medicine* 48 (2014): i18–i21. doi:10.1136/bjsports-2013-093223.

Kozir, L. Perry. "American College of Sports Medicine Current Comment: Alcohol and Athletic Performance." Accessed February 7, 2015. http://www.acsm.org/docs … alcoholandathleticperformance.pdf.

Kreider, Richard B., Colin D. Wilborn, Lem Taylor, Bill Campbell, Anthony L. Almada, Rick Collins, Mathew Cooke, et al. "International Society of Sports Nutrition Exercise and Sport Nutrition Review: Research and Recommnedations." *Journal of the International Society of Sports Nutrition* 7, no. 7 (2010). doi: 10.1186/1550-2783-7-7.

Larson, Nicole, Rich MacLehose, Jayne Fulkerson, Jerica Berge, Mary Sotry, and Dianne Neumark-Sztainer. "Eating Breakfast and Dinner Together as a Family: Associations with Sociodemographic Characteristics and Implications for Diet Quality and Weight Status." *Journal of the Academy of Nutrition and Dietetics* 113, no. 12 (2013): 1601–1609. doi:10.1016/j.and2013.08.011.

Lawrence, Glen D. "Dietary Fats and Health: Dietary Recommendations in the Context of Scientific Evidence." *Advances in Nutrition* 4, no. 3 (2013): 294–302. doi: 10.3945/an.113.003657.

Love, Page. "Nutrition Performance Diet Principles for Competitive Tennis." United States Tennis Association (USTA). Accessed February 8, 2015. http://www.usta.com/ … /119901_Nutrition_Performance_Diet_Principles_for_Competitive_Tennis/.

Love, Page. "Nutrition: Sports Supplements: Do They Enhance Tennis?" United States Tennis Association (USTA). Accessed February 8, 2015. www.usta.com/ ... /114733_Nutrition_Sports_Supplements_Do-They_Work.

Lukaski, Henry C., Emily Haymes, and Mitch Kanter. "American College of Sports Medicine Current Comment: Vitamin and Mineral Supplements and Exercise." https://www.acsm.org/ ... /vitaminandmineralsupplementsandexercise.pdf.

Lutz, Doris Jane. Interview by Grace Lee. 2013.

Mahan, Kathleen, Sylvia Escott-Stump, and Janice Raymond. *Krause's Food and the Nutrition Care Process*. 13th ed. Saint Louis: Saunders, 2013.

Mahoney, Caroline, Holly A. Taylor, Robin B. Kanarek, and Priscilla Samuel. "Effect of Breakfast Composition on Cognitive Processes in Elementary School Children." *Physiology and Behavior* 85 (2005): 635–645.

Maughan, Ron, and Louise Burke. *Handbook of Sports Medicine and Sports Science, Sports Nutrition*. Hoboken, NJ: Wiley-Blackwell, 2002.

May, Michelle. *Am I Hungry? What to Do When Diets Don't Work*. Phoenix: Nourish Publishers, 2004.

Mayo Clinic. "Hyponatremia." Reviewed May 28, 2014. http://www.mayoclinic.org/disease-conditions-/hyponatremia/basics/prevention/con-20031445.

McCulloch, Marsha. "Saturated Fat: No So Bad or Just Bad Science." *Today's Dietitian* 116, no. 11 (2014): 32.

McCormick, Teo. "Eating Disorders—The Coaches Role." United States Tennis Association. Accessed February 8, 2015. http://www.usta.com/Improve-Your-Game/Sport-Science /114717_Nutrition_Eating_Disorders_The_Coaches_Role/.

Miller, Margaret. *Enduring Words for the Athlete*. Columbus, OH: School Specialty Publishing, 2006.

Moeller, S. M., S. A. Fryhofer, A. J. Osbahr, and C. B. Robinowitz. "The Effects of High Fructose Corn Syrup." *Journal of the American College of Nutrition* 6 (2009): 619–626.

National Cancer Institute. "Alcohol and Cancer Risk." June 24, 2013. http://www.cancer.gov/cancertopics/factsheet/risk/alcohol.

National Cancer Institute. "Antioxidants and Cancer Prevention." Reviewed January 16, 2014. http://www.cancer.gov/topics/factsheets/antioxidants.

National Eating Disorder Association (NEDA). Accessed February 8, 2015. http://www.nationaleatingdisorder.org/educators-and-coaches.

National Foundation for Celiac Awareness. "Diagnosis of Non-Celiac Gluten Sensitivity." Last updated February 8, 2015. http://www.celiaccentral.org/non-celiac-gluten-sensitivity/testing-and-diagnosis/.

National Heart, Lung, and Blood Institute. "Body Mass Index." Accessed January 15, 2015. http://www.nhlbisupport.com/bmi/bmiinojs.htm.

National Heart, Lung, and Blood Institute/National Institutes of Health National Cholesterol Education Program. "ATP III At-A-Glance: Quick Desk Reference." Accessed February 16, 2015. http:// www.nhlbi.nih.gov /health-pro/guidelines / current/cholesterol-guidelines/quick-desk-reference-html.

National Heart, Lung, and Blood Institute. "Serving Sizes and Portions, Eat Right." Last updated September 30, 2013. http://www.nhlbi.nih.gov/health/public/heart/obesity/wecan/eat-right/distortion.htm.

National Institutes of Health/National Center for Complementary and Alternative Medicine. "Dietary Supplements and Diabetes." Last updated November 2013. http://www.nccam.nih/gov/health/diabetes/supplements.

National Institutes of Health/National Center for Complementary and Integrative Health. "Ephedra." Updated June 2013. https://www.nccih.nih.gov/health/ephedra.

National Institutes of Health, US National Library of Medicine. "Genetics Home Reference: Lactose Intolerance." Published May 4, 2015. Accessed May 12, 2015. http://www.ghr.nlm.gov/condition/lactose-intolerance

National Institutes of Health, Office of Dietary Supplements. "Dietary Supplement Fact Sheet: Vitamin E." Reviewed June 5, 2013. http://www.ods.od.nih.gov/factsheets/vitamin E-HealthProfessional.

National Institutes of Health, Office of Dietary Supplements. "Vitamin D Health Professional Fact Sheet." Reviewed November 10, 2014. http://www.ods.od.nih.gov/vitamin D-health professional.

National Institutes of Health, Office of Dietary Supplements. "Facts About Zinc." Reviewed June 5, 2013. http://www.ods.od.nih.gov/factsheets/zinc/healthprofessional/.

National Institutes of Health, Office of Dietary Supplements. "Dietary Supplements: What You Need to Know." Accessed February 12, 2014. http://www.ods.od.nih.gov/healthinformation/DS_whatyouneedtoknow.aspx.

National Institutes of Health, Office of Dietary Supplements. "Calcium—Dietary Supplement Fact Sheet." Accessed January 31, 2015. http://www.ods.od.nih.gov/factsheets/calciumhealthprofessional/.

National Institutes of Health. "What Is a Standard Drink?" National Institute on Alcohol Abuse and Alcoholism. Accessed March 7, 2015. http://www.niaaa.nih.gov/alcohol-health/overview-alcohol-consumption/standard-drink.

National Safety Foundation. "National Safety Foundation Consumer Information: Importance of Dietary Supplements." Accessed February 14, 2015. http://www.nsf.org/consumer/

dietarysupplements/dietarycertification.NSF    sport.com/
about.asps.

National Weight Control Registry. Accessed January 5, 2015.
http://www.nwcr.ws/.

Nattiv, Aurelia, Anne Loucks, Melinda Manore, Charlotte
Sanbour, Jorum Sundgot-Borgen, and Michelle Warren.
"American College of Sports Medicine Position Stand:
The Female Athlete Triad." *Medicine and Science in Sports
and Exercise* 39, no. 10 (2007): 1867–1882. doi: 10:1249/
mss.06013e318149f111.

Nebeling, Linda, Amy L. Yaroch, Jennifer Seymour, and Joel
Kimmons. "Still Not Enough: Can We Achieve Our Goals
for Americans to Eat More Fruits and Vegetables in the
Future?" *American Journal of Preventive Medicine* 32, no. 4
(2007): 354–355.

Nelson, Jennifer. "What is High Fructose Corn Syrup? What
Are the Health Concerns?" Nutrition and Healthy Eating:
Mayo Clinic. September 27, 2012. http://www.mayoclinic.
com/health/high-fructose-corn-syrup.

Nemet, Dan, and Alon Eliakim. "Pediatric Sports Nutrition: An
Update." *Current Opinion in Clinical Nutrition and Metabolic
Care, Pediatrics* 12, no. 3 (2009): 304–309. doi:10.1097/
MCO.0b013e32832a215b.

Oded, Bar-Or. "Nutrition for Child and Adolescent Athletes."
Gatorade Sports Science Institute Sports Science Exchange
#77. 2000. http://gssiweb.org/sports-science-exchange.

Oldways Preservation Trust/Whole Grains Council. Accessed
February 8, 2015. http://www.wholegrainscouncil.org/
whole-grain-stamp.

Olson, Eric D. "Bottled Water: Pure Drink or Pure Hype?"
*Natural Resources Defense Council.* 1999. Last revised July
15, 2013. Accessed January 21, 2015. http://www.nrdc.org /
water/drinking/bw/chap2.asp.

Organic Trade Association. http://www.ota.com.

Physicians Committee on Responsible Medicine. "PowerPlate." Accessed March 20, 2014. http://www.pcrm.org/images/ health/ppplate /EveryMealPowerPlate.,

Peltier, Sebastien L., Pierre-Marie Lepretre, Lore Metz, Gael Ennequin, Nicolas Aubineau, Jean-Francois Lescuyer, Martine Duclos, Thibault Brink, and Pascal Sirvent. "Effects of Pre-Exercise Endurance, and Recovery Designer Sports Drinks on Performance During Tennis Tournament Situation." *Journal of Strength and Conditioning Research* 27, no. 11 (2013): 3076–3083. doi: 10/1519/JSC.0b013e31828a4745.

Pluim, B. M., A. Ferraulti, F. Broekhof, M. Deutekom, A. Gotzmann, H. Kuipers, and K. Weber. "The Effect of Creatine Supplementation on Selected Factors of Tennis Specific Training." *British Journal of Sports Medicine* 40, no. 6 (2006): 507–512.

Portman, Robert, and Mark Kovacs. "Extend Practice by 15 Minutes for Nutritional Repair of Muscles." United States Professional Tennis Association (USPTA). Accessed March 8, 2015. http://www.tennis-health.com/Extendpracticeby15 minutesfornutritionalrepair/tabid/17/Default.aspx.

"Position of the Academy of Nutrition and Dietetics, Dietitians of Canada and the American College of Sports Medicine: Nutrition and Athletic Performance." *Journal of the Academy of Nutrition and Dietetics* 100, no. 12 (2000): 1543–1556.

Radak, Tim. "Confusing New Food Pyramid Misleads Consumers About Healthy Eating." Physicians Committee on Responsible Medicine. Accessed February 4, 2015. http://pcrm.org/ ... / disaster-by-design-confusing-new-food-pyramid.

Ranchordas, Mayur K., David Rogersion, Alan Ruddock, Sophie C. Killer, and Edward M. Winter. "Nutrition for Tennis: Practical Recommendations." *Journal of Sports Science and Medicine* 12, no. 2 (2013): 211–224.

Reedy, Jill, and Susan M. Krebs-Smith. "Dietary Sources of Energy, Solid Fats, and Added Sugars Among Children and

Adolescents in the United States." *Journal of the Academy of Nutrition and Dietetics* 110, no. 10 (2010): 1477–1484. doi: 10.1016/jada.2010.07.010.

Rolls, Barbara. *The Ultimate Volumetrics Diet: Smart, Simple Science-Based Strategies for Losing Weight and Keeping it Off.* New York: Harper Collins, 2005.

Rosenbloom, Christine A., and Ellen J. Coleman. *Academy of Nutrition and Dietetics Sports Nutrition: A Practice Manual For Professionals.* Chicago: Diana Faulhaber Publisher, 2012.

Rubio-Tapia, Alberto, Jonas Ludvigsson, Tricia Brantner, Joseph Murray, and James Everhart. "The Prevalence of Celiac Disease in the United States." *American Journal of Gastroenterology* 107 (2012): 1538.

Schaeffer, Juliean. "To Good Wine and Better Health—The Case for Moderate Wine Consumption." *Today's Dietitian* 13, no. 8 (2012): 32–35.

Schardt, David. "Coconut Oil." Center for Science in the Public Interest Nutrition Action Health Newsletter, June 2012. http://www.cspinet.org.nah/articles/coconut-oil.html.

Schardt, David. "Milking the Data." *Center for Science in the Public Interest—Nutrition Action Newsletter,* September 2005.

Seles, Monica. *Getting a Grip.* New York: Penguin Publishing, 2009.

Simpson, Michael, and Tom Howard. "Selecting and Effectively Using Hydration for Fitness." American College of Sports Medicine Consumer Information Committee, 2011. Accessed February 21, 2015. http://www.acsm.org/docs/ ... and-effectively-using-hydration-for-fitness.pdf.

Slining, M. M., and B. M. Popkin. "Trends in Intakes and Sources of Solid Fats and Added Sugars Among U.S. Children and Adolescents: 1994–2010." *Pediatric Obesity* 8, no. 4 (2013): 307–324. doi:10.1111/j.2047-6310.2013.00156.x.

Smith, Steve. Interview by Grace Lee. 2012.

Spano, Marie, and Chad Kersick. "Speeding Recovery: Nutrition and Supplementation for Exercise." *Today's Dietitian* 9, no. 9 (2007): 33–35.

Spriet, Lawrence, and Terry Graham. "American College of Sports Medicine Current Comment: Caffeine and Exercise Performance." Accessed January 21, 2015. http://www.acsm. org/docs/current-comments/caffeineandexercise.pdf.

Statista. "Non-Alcoholic Beverages and Soft Drinks in the United States." Accessed January 29, 2015. http://www. statista.com/ topics/1662/non-alcoholic-beverages-and-soft-drinks-in-the-United-States.

Stoler, Felicia D. "American College of Sports Medicine Current Comment. Childhood Obesity." Accessed October 15, 2014. http://www.acsm.org/docs /current … /childhoodobesity temp.pdf.

Tantamango-Bartley, Yessenia, Karen Jaceldo-Siegl, Jing Fan, and Gary Fraser. "Vegetarian Diets and the Incidence of Cancer in a Low-Risk Population." *Cancer Epidemiological Biomarkers and Prevention* 22, no. 2 (2013): 286–294. doi: 10.1158/1055-9965. EPI-12-1060.

Thiault Brink-Elfegoun, Ratel Sebastien, Pierre-Marie Lepretre, Lore Metz, Gael Ennequin, Eric Dore, Vincent Martin, David Bishop, Nicoloas Aubineau, Jean-Francois Lescuyer, Martine Duclos, Pascal Sirvent, and Sebastien L. Peltier. "Effects of Sports Drinks on the Maintenance of Physcial Performance During 3 Tennis Matches: A Randomized Controlled Study." *Journal of the International Society of Sports Nutrition* 11, no. 46 (2014). doi:10.1186/s12970-014-0046-7.

United States Department of Agriculture. "Healthy, Hunger-Free Kids Act." Last modified March 3, 2014. http://www.fns. usda.gov/school-meals/healthy-hunger-free-kids-act.

United States Department of Agriculture. "MyPlate." http:// www.choosemyplate.gov/.

United States Department of Agriculture. "National Nutrient Database for Standard Reference, Release 27." Last modified December 7, 2011. http://www.ndb.nal.usda.gov/ndb/nutrients.

United States Department of Agriculture. "Certified Organic Seal." Accessed January 30, 2015. http://www.ams.usda.gov/AMSv1.0/getfile.

United States Department of Agriculture. "Smart Snacks in School." Accessed January 12, 2015. http://www.fns.usda.gov/healthierschoolday/tools-schools-focusing-smart-snacks.

United States Department of Agriculture. "2010 Dietary Guidelines for Americans." Accessed January 11, 2015. http://www.health.gov/dietary guidelines/dga2010.

United States Department of Agriculture, National Nutrient Database for Standard Reference. "Fiber Content of Foods, Release 17." 2004. http://www.nal.usda.gov/fnic/foodcomp.

United States Pharmacopeia. "United States Pharmacopeia Verified Dietary Supplements." Accessed February 8, 2015. http://www.usp.org/usp-verification-services/usp-verified-dietary-supplements.

United States Tennis Association. "Nutrition: Key Pointers for Tennis." Accessed February 8, 2015. http://www.usta.com/Improve-Your-Game/Sport Science/114722_Nutrition_Key_Pointers_for_Tennis/.

United States Tennis Association. "Post-Match Nutrition." Accessed February 8, 2015. http://www.usta.com/Improve-Your-Game/Sport-Science/119902_Nutrition_PostMatch_Nutrition/.

University of California, Berkeley. "The Sunny Side of Eggs." May 1, 2013. Accessed January 21, 2014. http://www.berkeleywellness.com/healthy/eating/nutrition/article/sunny-side-eggs.

Vergauwen, Lieven, Fred Brouns, and Peter Hespel. "Carbohydrate Supplementation Improves Stroke Performance in Tennis."

*Journal of Sports Science and Medicine* 30, no. 8 (1998): 1289–1295.

Volek, J. S., B. M. Volk, L. J. Kunces, B. R. Kupchak, D. J. Freidenriech, J. C. Aristizabal, C. Saenz, et al. "Whey Protein Supplementation During Resistance Training Augments Lean Body Mass." *Journal of the American College of Nutrition*, 32, no. 2 (2013): 122-135. doi: 10.1080/07315724.2013/793580.

Walsh, Brian. "Don't Blame Fat." *Time*, June 23, 2014.

Webb, Denise. "Athletes and Protein Intake." *Today's Dietitian* 16, no. 6 (2014): 22–25.

White, J. S. "Straight Talk About High Fructose Corn Syrup: What It Is and What It Ain't." *American Journal of Clinical Nutrition* 88, no. 6 (2008): 1716S–1721S. doi: 10.3945/ajcn.2008.25825B.

Willett, Gina. "Scientific Advances Regarding Sugar, Salt and Fat." 2nd ed. "Institute of Natural Resources Home Study 2630." March 2014.

Willett, W., F. Sacks, and M. Stampfer. "Dietary Fat and Heart Disease Is Seriously Misleading." Harvard University. March 19, 2014. http://www. hsph.harvard.edu/ … / dietary-fat-and-heart-disease.

World Anti-Doping Agency (WADA). Accessed February 8, 2015. http.//www.wada-ama.org/.

World's Healthiest Foods. Accessed February 8, 2015. http:// www.whfoods.com /genpage.

Wu, Ching-Lin, Mu-Shin Shih, Chia-Cheng Yang, Ming-Hsiang Huang, and Chen-Kang Chang. "Sodium Bicarbonate Supplementation Prevents Skilled Tennis Performance Decline After a Simulated Match." *Journal of the International Society of Sports Nutrition* 7, no. 33 (2010). doi:10.1186/1550-2783-7-33.

Xu, Jiaquan, Kenneth D. Kochanek, Sherry L. Murphy, and Elizabeth Arias. Center for Disease Control and Prevention. "Mortality in the United States, 2012." National Center for

Health Statistics Data Brief, no. 168. October 2014. http://www.cdc.gov/nchs/databrief/db168.pdf.

Yetley, Elizabeth A. "Multivitamin and Multimineral Dietary Supplements: Definitions, Characterization, Bioavailability and Drug Interactions." *The American Journal of Clinical Nutrition* 85, suppl (2007): 269S–276S.

Youbar—Custom Energy Bars. http://www. youbars.com. Accessed March 8, 2015.

Yusuf, S., G. Dagenais, J. Pogue, J. Bosch, and P. Sleight. "Vitamin E Supplementation and Cardiovascular Events in High-Risk Patients. The Heart Outcomes Prevention Evaluation (HOPE) Study Investigators." *The New England Journal of Medicine* 342, no. 3 (2000): 154–160. doi:10.1056/NEJM200001203420302.

Zemel, Michael B. "Role of Calcium and Dairy Products in Energy Partitioning and Weight Management." *American Journal of Clinical Nutrition* 79, no. 5 (2004): 907S–912S.

# NOTES

## INTRODUCTION

1   Jimmy Arias, interview by Grace Lee, 2014.
2   Nick Bollettieri, interview by Grace Lee, 2012, 2015.
3   Ibid.
4   Doris Jane Lutz, interview by Grace Lee, 2013.

## CHAPTER 1

5   United States Department of Agriculture (USDA), "2010 Dietary Guidelines for Americans," accessed January 11, 2015, http://www. health.gov/dietaryguidelines/dga2010.
6   "Adult Obesity Facts," Center for Disease Control and Prevention, last reviewed September 9, 2014, http://www.cdc.gov/obesity/date/adult. html.
7   Jiaquan Xu et al., "Mortality in the United States," Center for Disease Control and Prevention, no. 168, October 2014.
8   "Adult Obesity Facts."
9   "ChooseMyPlate.gov," United States Department of Agriculture, accessed February 4, 2015, http://www.choosemyplate.gov/.
10  Tim Radak, "Confusing New Food Pyramid Misleads Consumers About Healthy Eating," Physicians Committee on Responsible Medicine (PCRM), accessed February 4, 2015, http://www. pcrm. org/ … /disaster-by-design-confusing-new-food-pyramid.
11  "Fruits and Vegetables for Health," World Health Organization, accessed February 4, 2015, http://www.who.int/dietphysicalactivity/ publications /fruit_vegetables_report.pdf.
12  "ChooseMyPlate.gov."

13  "Vegetables and Fruits: Get Plenty Every Day," Harvard School of Public Health, accessed March 8, 2015, http://www. hsph.harvard.edu/nutritionsource/vegetables-full story.

14  W. J. Craig and A. R. Mangels, "Position of the Academy of Nutrition and Dietetics: Vegetarian Diets," *Journal of the Academy of Nutrition and Dietetics* 109, no. 7 (2009): 1266.

15  "Powerplate," Physician's Committee on Responsible Medicine, accessed March 20, 2014, http://www.pcrm.org/health /diets/power-plate.

16  "State Indicator Report on Fruits and Vegetables," Center for Disease Control and Prevention, accessed January 15, 2015, http://www.cdc.gov/nutrition/downloads/StateIndicatorReport2009.pdf.

17  Ibid.

18  "Organic Agriculture," US Department of Agriculture, updated January 9, 2015, http://www.usda.gov/organic-agriculture.html.

19  "EWG's 2014 Shopper's Guide to Pesticides in Produce," Environmental Working Group, Executive Summary, reviewed April 2014, http://www.ewg.org/foodnews/summary.php.

20  "American Academy of Pediatrics Weighs in for the First Time on Organic Foods for Children," Press Release, American Academy of Pediatrics, October 22, 2012, http://www.aap.org/en-us/about-the-aap/aap-press-room.

21  "Certified Organic Seal," United States Department of Agriculture, accessed January 30, 2015, http://www.ams.usda.gov/AMSv1.0/getfile.

22  Ibid.

23  Ibid.

24  Marcin Baranski et al., "Higher Antioxidant and Lower Cadmium Concentrations and Lower Incidence of Pesticide Residues in Organically Grown Crops: A Systemic Literature Meta-Analysis," *British Journal of Nutrition* 125, no. 5 (2014): 794–811, doi:10.1017/S00007114514001366.Epub2014Jun26.

25  Kathleen Mahan, Sylvia Escott-Stump, and Janice Raymond. *Krause's Food and Nutrition Care Process*, 13th ed. (Philadelphia: Saunders, 2013).

26  "Nutrition Fact Sheet: The Sunny Side of Vitamin D," Academy of Nutrition and Dietetics, Sports, Cardiovascular and Nutrition Practice Group, http://www.eatright.org.

27  "Dietary Reference Intakes for Calcium and Vitamin D Report Brief," Institute of Medicine, posted November 30, 2010, http://www.iom.

edu/Reports/2010/Dietary-Reference-Intakes-for-Calcium-and-Vitamin-D.aspx.

28  "Vitamin D Health Professional Fact Sheet," Office of Dietary Supplements, National Institutes of Health, reviewed November 10, 2014, http://www.ods.od.nih.gov/vitamin D-health professional.

29  "Dietary Reference Intakes for Calcium and Vitamin D."

30  "Genetics Home Reference: Lactose Intolerance," National Institutes of Health, US National Library of Medicine, published May 4, 2015, accessed May 12, 2015, http://ghr.nlm.gov/condition / lactose-intolerance.

31  "National Nutrient Database for Standard Reference, Release 27," United States Department of Agriculture, last modified December 12, 2011, http://www.ndb.nal.usda.gov/.

32  "We Can! Eat Right," National Heart, Lung, and Blood Institute, updated September 13, 2013, http://www.nhlbi.nih.gov /health/ public/obesity/wecan/eat-right/distortion.htm.

33  "Portion Sizes Twenty Years Ago and Today," National Heart, Lung, and Blood Institute, updated September 13, 2013, http://www.nhlbi. nih.gov/health/public/obesity/wecan/eat-right/distortion.htm.

34  Barbara Rolls, *The Ultimate Volumetrics Diet: Smart Simple Science-based Strategies for Losing Weight and Keeping it Off* (New York: Harper Collins, 2005).

35  Yessenia Tantamango-Bartley et al., "Vegetarian Diets and the Incidence of Cancer in a Low-Risk Population," *Cancer Epidemiology Biomarkers and Prevention* 22, no. 2 (2013): 286, doi: 10.1158/1055-9965.EPI-12-1060.

36  "Harvard Healthy Eating Plate," Harvard University School of Public Health, accessed February 5, 2015, http://www.health.harvard.edu/ plate/health-heating-plate.

## CHAPTER 2

37  Richard Kreider et al., "International Society of Sports Nutrition Exercise and Sports Nutrition Review: Research and Recommendations," *Journal of the International Society of Sports Nutrition* 7, no. 7 (2010), doi:10.1186/1550-2783-7-7.

38  Michael F. Holick, "Resurrection of Vitamin D Deficiency and Rickets," *Journal of Clinical Investigation* 116, no. 8 (2006): 2062.

39  Elizabeth A. Yetley, "Multivitamin and Multimineral Dietary Supplements: Definitions, Characterization, Bioavailability and Drug Interactions," *The American Journal of Clinical Nutrition,* 85, supp (2007): 269S–276S.

40  "Dietary Supplements and Diabetes," National Institutes of Health (NIH)/National Center for Complementary and Alternative Medicine, last updated November 2013, http://www.nccam.nih.gov/health/diabetes/supplements.

41  Henry C. Lukaski, Emily Haymes, and Mitch Kanter. "American College of Sports Medicine Current Comment: Vitamin and Mineral Supplements and Exercise," accessed February 14, 2015, http://www.acsm.org./ … /vitaminandmineralsupplementsandexercise.pdf.

42  Kreider et al., "Exercise and Sports Nutrition Review."

43  Andrew M. Jones, "Dietary Nitrate: The New Magic Bullet?" Gatorade Sports Science Institute Sports Science Exchange #106, accessed January 12, 2015, http://www.gssiweb.org /sports-science-exchange.

44  World Anti-Doping Association (WADA), accessed February 8, 2015, http://www.wada-ama.org/.

45  "International Tennis Foundation Anti-Doping Programme," International Tennis Foundation, accessed February 8, 2015, http: // www.itftennis.com/anti-doping.

46  Ibid.

47  "World Anti-Doping Association Mission Statement," World Anti-Doping Association, accessed February 8, 2015, http://www.wada-ama.org/.

48  "United States Pharmacopeia Verified Dietary Supplements," United States Pharmacopeia, accessed February 8, 2015, http://www. usp.org/usp-verification-services/usp-verified-dietary-supplements.

49  "National Safety Foundation Consumer Information: Importance of Dietary Supplements," National Safety Foundation accessed February 14, 2015, http://www.nsf.org/consumer/dietarysupplements/dietarycertification.NSF sport.com/about.asps.

50  "Tips for Dietary Supplement Users," Food and Drug Administration, last updated April 23, 2014, http://www.fda.gov/Food/DietarySupplements/UsingDietarySupplements.

51  National Institutes of Health, http://www.ods.od.nih.gov.

52  American College of Sports Medicine, "Position Stand: Nutrition and Athletic Performance," *Medicine and Science in Sports and Exercise* 38, no. 3 (2009): 709–731.

53  Kreider et al., "Exercise and Sport Nutrition Review."

54  B. M. Pluim et al., "The Effects of Creatine Supplementation on Selected Factors of Tennis Specific Training," *British Journal of Sports Medicine* 40, no. 6 (2006): 507–512.

55  Ibid.

56  Tiffany Dabek Davis, interview, October 21, 2014.

57  American College of Sports Medicine, "Position Stand: Nutrition and Athletic Performance."

58  Lawrence L. Spreit and Terry E. Graham, "American College of Sports Medicine Current Comment—Caffeine and Exercise Performance," accessed January 21, 2015, http://www.acsm.org /docs/current-comments/caffeineandexercise.pdf.

59  Ibid.

60  Damian Farrow, "Caffeine, Carbohydrate and Cooling Use During Prolonged Simulated Tennis," *International Journal of Sports Physiology and Performance* 2, no. 4 (2008): 423–438.

61  Spreit, "Caffeine and Exercise Performance."

62  Ching-Lin Wu et al., "Sodium Bicarbonate Supplementation Prevents Skilled Tennis Performance Decline After a Simulated Match," *Journal of the International Society of Sports Nutrition* 7, no. 33 (2010), doi: 10.1186/1150-2783-7-33.

63  W. Larry Kenney, Jack H. Wilmore, and David L. Costill. *Physiology of Sport and Exercise*, 5th ed. (Champaign, IL: Human Kinetics, 2012).

64  Bill Campbell et al., "International Society of Sports Nutrition and Position Stand: Protein and Exercise," *Journal of the International Society of Sports Nutrition* 4, no. 8 (2007), doi:10.1185/1150-2783-4-8.

65  American College of Sports Medicine, "Position Stand: Nutrition and Athletic Performance."

66  Ibid.

67  "Ephedra," National Institutes of Health, National Center for Complementary and Integrative Health, updated June 2013, https://www.nccih.nih.gov/health/ephedra.

68  "International Tennis Foundation Anti-Doping Programme."

69  Ibid.

70  S. Yusuf et al., "Vitamin E Supplementation and Cardiovascular Events in High-Risk Patients. The Heart Outcomes Prevention Evaluation Study Investigators," *Journal of the American Medical Association* 342, no. 3 (2000): 154, doi: 10.1056 /NEJM200001203420302.

71  "Antioxidants and Cancer Prevention," National Cancer Institute, reviewed January 16, 2014, http://www.cancer.gov/topics/factsheets/antioxidants.

72  http://www.fda.gov/Food/GuidanceRegulation  /  GuidanceDocumentsRegulatoryInformation/LabelingNutrition/ucm385663, Feb 27, 2014.

## CHAPTER 3

73  Margo A. Denke, "Metabolic Effects of High-Protein, Low-Carbohydrate Diets," *American Journal of Cardiology* 88 (2001): 59–61.

74  "Livestock a Major Threat to the Environment," Food and Agricultural Organization Newsroom, accessed January 28, 2015, www.fao.org/newsroom /en/news/2006/1000448 /index.html.

75  Richard B. Kreider et al., "International Society of Sports Nutrition Exercise and Sport Nutrition Review: Research and Recommendations," 10.

76  Bill Campbell et al., "International Society of Sports Nutrition Position Stand: Protein and Exercise," *Journal of the International Society of Sports* Nutrition 4, no. 8 (2007), doi:10.1186/1550-2783-4-8.

77  American College of Sports Medicine, "Nutrition and Athletic Performance," *Medicine and Science in Sports and Exercise* 41, no. 3 (2009): 718.

78  Campbell et al., "Position Stand: Protein and Exercise."

79  Ibid.

80  Mayur R. Ranchordas et al., "Nutrition for Tennis: Practical Recommendations," *Journal of Sports Science and Medicine* 12, no. 2 (2013): 211-224.

81  Nick Bollettieri, interview by Grace Lee, 2012, 2015.

82  Dana Gunders, "Wasted: How America is Losing Up to 40 Percent of Its Food from Farm to Fork to Landfill, Natural Resources Defense Council (NRDC), Issue Paper, August 2012, IP:12-06-B, http://www.nrdc.org/food/files/wasted-food-ip.pdf.

83  Shersten Killip, John M. Bennett, and Mara D. Chambers, "Iron Deficiency Anemia," *American Family Physician* 75, no. 5, (2007): 671, www.aafp.org/afp/2013/0115 /p98.html.

84  Susan M. Kleiner, "The Role of Red Meat in the Athlete's Diet," Gatorade Sports Science Institute Sports Science Exchange #58 8, no. 5 (1995), https://www.gssiweb.org/en/sports-science-exchange.

85 National Institutes of Health, Office of Dietary Supplements. "Facts About Zinc," reviewed June 5, 2013, http://www.ods.od.nih.gov/factsheets/zinc/healthprofessional/.

86 Ibid.

87 Alberto Rubio-Tapia et al., "The Prevalence of Celiac Disease in the United States," *American Journal of Gastroenterology* 107 (2012): 1538.

88 "Diagnosis of Non-Celiac Gluten Sensitivity," National Foundation for Celiac Awareness, last updated February 8, 2015, http://www.celiaccentral.org/non-celiac-gluten-sensitivity/testing-and-diagnosis/.

89 Chad Kerksick et al., "International Society of Sports Nutrition Position Stand: Nutrient Timing," *Journal of the International Society of Sports Nutrition* 5, no. 17 (2008), doi: 10.1186/1550-2783-5-17.

90 Jay R. Hoffman and Michael J. Flavo, "Protein-Which Is Best?" International Society of Sports Nutrition Symposium, June 2005, *Journal of Sports Science and Medicine* 3 (2004): 118–130.

## CHAPTER 4

91 Glen D. Lawrence, "Dietary Fats and Health: Dietary Recommendations in the Context of Scientific Evidence," *Advances in Nutrition* 4 (2013): 294–295, doi: 10.3945/an.113.003657.

92 "Adult Treatment Plan (ATP) III At-A-Glance: Quick Desk Reference," National Heart Lung and Blood Institute/National Institutes of Health/National Cholesterol Education Program, accessed February 16, 2015, http://www.nhlbi.nih.gov/health-pro/guidelines /current/cholesterol-guidelines/quick-desk-reference-html.

93 R. Chowdury et al., "Association of Dietary, Circulating and Supplement Fatty Acids with Coronary Risk: A Systemic Review and Meta-Analysis. *Annals of Internal Medicine* 160, no. 6 (2014): 398, doi: 10.7326/M13-1788.

94 David Schardt, "Coconut Oil," Center for Science in the Public Interest Nutrition Action Health Letter, June 2012, http://www.cspinet.org.nah/articles/coconut-oil.thml. Thomas Brenna is quoted in this article.

95 "FDA Takes Steps to Further Reduce Trans Fat in Processed Foods," Food and Drug Administration (FDA), May 14, 2014, http://www.fda.gov/ForConsumers/ConsumerUpdates /ucm372915.htm.

96 Ibid.

97 Ramon Estruch et al., "Primary Prevention of Cardiovascular Disease with a Mediterranean Diet," *New England Journal of Medicine* 368, no. 14 (2013): 1279.

98 Ibid., 1297.

99 Toby Amidor, "Clean Eating," *Today's Dietitian* 15, no. 5 (May 2013): 10.

100 "Adult Treatment Plan (ATP) III At-A-Glance: Quick Desk Reference."

101 Mary Franz, "Nutrition, Inflammation and Disease," *Today's Dietitian* 16, no. 2 (2014): 44, http://www.todaysdietitian.com/pdf/courses / FranzInflammation.pdf.

102 Ibid.

103 Ibid.

104 "The Sunny Side of Eggs-Berkeley Wellness," University of California–Berkeley, last reviewed May 1, 2013, http://www.berkeley wellness. com/healthy-eating/.../sunny-side-eggs.

105 "Proposed Changes to the Nutrition Facts Label," Food and Drug Administration, last updated August 1, 2014, http://www.fda.gov/Food/ GuidanceRegulation /GuidanceDocumentsRegulatoryInformation/ LabelingNutrition/ucm385663.htm.

## CHAPTER 5

106 Gina Willett, "Scientific Advances Regarding Sugar, Salt and Fat," 2nd ed., Institute of Natural Resources, Home Study 2630, March 2014.

107 "Glycemic Index and Diabetes," American Diabetes Association, last modified March 14, 2014, http://www.diabetes.org/glycemic- index-and-diabetes.html.

108 "Health Gains from Whole Grains," Harvard University School of Public Health, accessed February 8, 2015, http://www.hsph.harvard. edu/nutritionsource/health-gains-from-whole-grains/.

109 "Using the Nutrition Facts Food Label," Food and Drug Administration, accessed January 25, 2015, http://www.fda.gov/ downloads/Food/ResourcesForYou/Consumers/UCM275396.pdf.

110 Lindsey Getz, "Deciphering Whole Grain Food Labels—Separating Fact from Fiction," *Today's Dietitian* 14, no. 6 (2012): 44.

111 "Whole Grain Stamp," Oldways Preservation Trust / Whole Grains Council, accessed February 8, 2015, http://www.wholegrainscouncil. org/whole-grain-stamp.

112 Ibid.

113 "Dietary Reference Intakes: Vitamins," Institute of Medicine, last updated October 12, 2014, http://www.iom.edu/-/media/Files/Activity%20Files/Nutrition/DRIs/DRI.

114 US Department of Agriculture National Database for Standard Reference, Release 27, last modified December 12, 2011, http://www.ndb.nal.usda.gov/.

115 "Launch of the International Year of Quinoa," Food and Agricultural Organization, 2013, http://www.fao.org/quinoa-2013/en/.

116 Christine A. Rosenbloom and Ellen Coleman, *Sports Nutrition—A Practice Manual for Professionals*, 5th ed. (Chicago: Diana Faulhaber Publisher, 2013), 5–9.

117 Ibid., 7.

118 American College of Sports Nutrition, "Position Stand: Nutrition and Athletic Performance," *Medicine and Science in Sports and Exercise* 41, no. 3 (2009): 709–731.

119 Ibid.

120 Mayur R. Ranchordas et al., "Nutrition for Tennis: Practical Recommendations," *Journal of Sports Science and Medicine* 12, no. 2 (2013): 211–224.

121 Ibid.

122 Nancy Clark, *Nancy Clark's Sports Nutrition Guidebook*, 5th ed. (Champaign, IL: Human Kinetics, 2014), 129.

123 "Glycemic Index and Diabetes," American Diabetes Association, last modified March 14, 2014, http://www.diabetes.org/glycemic-index-and-diabetes.html.

124 Ibid.

125 Ibid.

126 Chad Kerksick et al., "International Society of Sports Nutrition Position Stand: Nutrient Timing," *Journal of the International Society of Sports Nutrition* 5, no. 17 (2008).

127 Rosenbloom, *Sports Nutrition—A Practice Manual for Professionals*, 5th ed., 18.

128 Ranchordas, "Nutrition for Tennis," 211–224.

129 "Nutrition for Tennis," International Tennis Foundation Coaches Education Programme Level 2, February 12, 2007, http://www.en.coachingitftennis.com/media/113855/13855.pdf.

130 Asker Jeukendrup, "Multiple Transportable Carbohydrates and Their Benefits," Gatorade Sports Science Institute Sports Science Exchange #108, http://www.gssiweb.org/sports-science-exchange.

131 Ibid.

## CHAPTER 6

132 Steve Smith, interview by Grace Lee, 2012.

133 "Adult Obesity Facts," Center for Disease Control and Prevention (CDC), last reviewed September 9, 2014, http://www.cdc.gov /obesity/ data/adult.html.

134 National Heart Lung and Blood Institute, "Body Mass Index," accessed January 15, 2015, http://www.nhlbisupport.com /bmi/bmiinojs.htm.

135 Kathleen Mahan and Sylvia Escott-Stump, *Krause's Food and the Nutrition Care Process*, 13th ed. (Saint Louis: Saunders, 2013).

136 Michelle May, *Am I Hungry: What to Do When Diets Don't Work* (Phoenix: Nourish Publishers, 2004), 25.

137 Ibid, 31.

138 Ibid, 33.

139 Ibid, 30.

140 Susan Albers, "Mindful Eating Plate," accessed November 18, 2014, http://www.eatingmindfully.com.

141 Monica Seles, *Getting a Grip* (New York: Penguin Publishing, 2009).

142 *Diagnostic and Statistical Manual of Mental Disorders*, 5th ed. (Washington, DC: American Psychiatric Association, 2013).

143 National Eating Disorders Association (NEDA), accessed February 8, 2015, http://www.nationaleatingdisorder.org/educators-and-coaches.

144 American College of Sports Medicine, Current Comment: Eating Disorders, accessed January 25, 2015, http://www.acsm.org/docs / current-comments/eatingdisorders.pdf.

145 National Eating Disorders Association (NEDA), accessed February 8, 2015, http://www.nationaleatingdisorder.org/educators-and-coaches.

146 Academy of Nutrition and Dietetics, "The Female Athlete Triad," January 2010, accessed February 15, 2015, http://www.scandpg.org / sports-nutrition/sports-nutrition-fact-sheets/.

147 Aurelia Nattiv et al., "American College of Sports Medicine Position Stand: Female Athlete Triad," *Medicine in Sports Science and Exercise* 39, no. 10 (2007): 1867.

148 Nicole Larson et al., "Eating Breakfast and Dinner Together as a Family: Associations with Sociodemographic Characteristics and Implications for Diet Quality and Weight Status," *Journal of the Academy of Nutrition and Dietetics* 13, no. 2 (2013): 1601, doi: http:// dx.doi.org/10.1016/j.and2013.08.011.

149 Ibid.

150 Alexa Holyand, Louise Dye and Clare Lawton, "A Systemic Review of the Effect of Breakfast on Cognitive Performance of Children and Adolescents," *Nutrition Research Reviews* 22 (2009): 220–243, doi: 10.1017/S0954422409990175.

151 Academy of Nutrition and Dietetics, Fad Diet Timeline, accessed January 25, 2015, http://www.eatright.org/nnm/games /timeline / index.html.

152 National Weight Control Registry, accessed January 5, 2015, http:// www.nwcr.ws/.

153 Ibid.

## CHAPTER 7

154 American College of Sports Medicine Position Stand, "Exercise and Fluid Replacement," *Medicine and Science in Sports and Exercise* 39, no. 2 (2007): 377–390.

155 Ibid.

156 Ibid.

157 Ibid.

158 Tomoko Ichinose-Kuwahara, Yoshimitsu Inoue, Yoshiko Iseki, Sachi Hara, Yukio Ogura, and Narihiko Kondo, "Sex Differences on the Effects of Physical Training on Sweat Gland Responses During a Graded Exercise," *Experimental Physiology* 19, no. 10 (2010): 1026, doi: 10:1113/expphysiol.2010.053710.

159 American College of Sports Medicine Position Stand, "Exercise and Fluid Replacement," 377-390.

160 Michael Simpson and Tom Howard, "Selecting and Effectively Using Hydration for Fitness," American College of Sports Medicine, Consumer Information Committee, 2011, accessed February 21, 2015, http://www.acsm.org/docs/ ... and-effectively-using-hydration-for-fitness.pdf.

161 American College of Sports Medicine, "Exercise and Fluid Replacement," 377–390.

162 Mayur R. Ranchordas et al., "Nutrition for Tennis: Practical Recommendations," *Journal of Sports Science and Medicine* 12, no. 2 (2013): 211–224.

163 Eric D. Olson, "Bottled Water: Pure Drink or Pure Hype?" Natural Resources Defense Council, 1999, last revised July 15, 2013, accessed January 21, 2015, http://www.nrdc.org/water/drinking/bw/chap2.asp.

164 "Bottled Water Sales and Consumption Projected to Increase in 2014, Expected to be the Number One Packaged Drink by 2016," American Bottled Water Association, Press Release, December 4, 2014, accessed May 13, 2015, http://www.bottledwater.org/bottled-water-sales-and-consumption-projected-increase-2014-expected-to-be-number-one-packaged-drink.

165 Olson, "Bottled Water: Pure Drink or Pure Hype?"

166 American College of Sports Medicine, "Selecting and Effectively Using Sports Drinks, Carbohydrate Gels and Energy Bars," American College of Sports Medicine, Consumer Information Committee, 2011, accessed February 21, 2015, http://www.acsm.org/docs/brochures / selecting-and-effectively-using-sports-drinks-carbohydrate-gels-and-energy-bars.

167 American College of Sports Medicine, "Exercise and Fluid Replacement," 377–390.

168 Asker Jeukendrup, "Multiple Transportable Carbohydrates and Their Benefits," Gatorade Sports Science Institute Sports Science Exchange #108, accessed January 25, 2015.

169 Chad Kerksick et al., "International Society of Sports Nutrition Position Stand: Nutrient Timing," *Journal of the International Society of Sports Nutrition* 5, no. 17, (2008), doi: 10.1186/1550-2783-5-17.

170 Ibid.

171 Bill Campbell, "International Society of Sports Nutrition Position Stand: Energy Drinks," *Journal of the Society of International Sports Nutrition* 10, no. 1 (2013), doi: 10.1186/1550-2783-10-1

172 Lawrence L. Spriet and Terry E. Graham, American College of Sports Medicine, "Current Comment: Caffeine and Exercise Performance," accessed January 20, 2015, http://www.acsm.org /docs/current-comments/caffeineandexercise.pdf.

173 Ibid.

174 Ibid.

175 Richard Kreider et al., "International Society of Sports Nutrition Exercise and Sports Nutrition Review: Research and

Recommendations," *Journal of the International Society of Sports Nutrition* 7, no. 7 (2010).

176 Spriet and Graham, "Current Comment: Caffeine and Exercise Performance."

177 Kreider et al., "International Society of Sports Nutrition Exercise and Sports Nutrition Review: Research and Recommendations."

178 "Caffeine Content of Various Food and Beverages," Center for Science in the Public Interest, November 2014, http: //www.cspinet.org/new/cafchart.

179 Spriet and Graham, "Current Comment: Caffeine and Exercise Performance."

180 Nancy Clark, *Nancy Clark's Sports Nutrition Guidebook*, 5th ed. (Champaign, IL: Human Kinetics, 2014), 170.

181 Douglas S. Kalman et al., "Comparison of Coconut Water and a Carbohydrate-Electrolyte Sport Drink on Measures of Hydration and Physical Performance on Exercise-trained Men," *Journal of the International Society of Sports Nutrition* 9, no. 1 (2012), doi: 10.1186/1550-27839-9-1.

182 "Non-Alcoholic Beverages and Soft Drinks," Statista, accessed January 29, 2015, http://www.statista.com/topics/non-alcoholic-beverages-and-soft-drinks.

183 S. M. Moeller et al., "The Effects of High Fructose Corn Syrup," *Journal of the American College of Nutrition* 28, no. 6 (2009): 619–626.

184 Ibid., 619.

185 Ibid., 619.

186 Academy of Nutrition and Dietetics, Position Paper, "Use of Nutritive and Non-Nutritive Sweeteners," *Journal of the Academy of Nutrition and Dietetics* 112, no. 5 (2012): 749.

187 J. S. White, "Straight Talk About High Fructose Corn Syrup: What It Is and What It Ain't," *American Journal of Clinical Nutrition* 88, no. 6 (2008): 1716S–1721S, doi:10:3945/ajcn.2008.25825B.

188 Center for Disease Control and Prevention, "Alcohol and Public Health," http://www. cdc.gov/ … /2012.

189 "Alcohol and Cancer Risk," National Cancer Institute, June 24, 2013, http://www.cancer.gov/cancertopics /factsheet/risk/alcohol.

190 Juliean Schaeffer, "To Good Wine and Better Health—The Case for Moderate Wine Consumption," *Today's Dietitian* 13, no. 8 (2011): 32–35.

191 Michael Bergeron, "Heat and Hydration in Young Tennis Players," American College of Sports Medicine Current Comment, accessed January 28, 2015, http://www.acsm.org/docs/current-comments / heatandhydration.pdf.

192 Ibid.

193 American College of Sports Medicine, "Nutrition and Athletic Performance," *Medicine and Science in Sports and Exercise* 41, no. 3 (2009): 709–731.

194 Bergeron, "Heat and Hydration."

195 "Hyponatremia," Mayo Clinic, reviewed May 28, 2014, http://www. mayoclinic.org /diseases-conditions/hyponatremia/basics/prevention/ com-20031445.

196 Bergeron, "Heat and Hydration."

197 American College of Sports Medicine, "Exercise and Fluid Replacement."

198 Ranchordas, "Nutrition for Tennis: Practical Recommendations," 211–224.

199 Bergeron, "Heat and Hydration."

200 American College of Sports Medicine, "Exercise and Fluid Replacement," 377–390.

## CHAPTER 8

201 Novak Djokovic, *Serve to Win: The 14-Day Gluten-Free Plan for Physical and Mental Excellence* (New York: Zinc Ink, 2013), xxiv.

202 J. S. Volek, B. M. Volk, L. J. Kunces, B. R. Kupchak, D. J. Freidenriech, J. C. Aristizabal, C. Saenz, et al., "Whey Protein Supplementation During Resistance Training Augments Lean Body Mass," *Journal of the American College of Nutrition*, 32, no. 2 (2013): 122-135, doi: 10.1080/07315724.2013/793580.

203 Mayur R. Ranchordas et al., "Nutrition for Tennis: Practical Recommendations," *Journal of Sports Science and Medicine* 12, no. 2 (2013): 211–224.

## CHAPTER 9

204 Steve Smith, interview by Grace Lee, 2012, and correspondence, 2015.

205 Steve Smith, interview by Grace Lee, 2012, and correspondence, 2015.

206 Nick Bollettieri, interview by Grace Lee, 2012, and correspondence, 2015.

207 Meghan M. Slining and Barry M. Popkin, "Trends in Intakes and Sources of Solid Fats and Added Sugars Among Children and Adolescents: 1994–2010," *Pediatric Obesity* 8, no. 4 (2013): 307–324, doi: 10.1111/j.2047-6310.2013.00156.x.

208 Jill Reedy and Susan Krebs-Smith, "Dietary Sources of Energy, Solid Fats, and Added Sugars Among Children and Adolescents in the United States," *Journal of the Academy of Nutrition and Dietetics* 110, no. 10 (2010): 1477, doi: 10.1016/jada.2010.07.010.

209 "Childhood Obesity Facts," Center for Disease Control and Prevention last modified December 11, 2014, http://www.cdc.gov/healthyyouth / obesity/fact.htm.

210 Institute of Natural Resources, "Food Habits, Cravings and Emotions," seminar, presented by Michelle Albers, Bradenton, Florida, March 2014.

211 Ibid.

212 Bar-or Oded, "Nutrition For Child and Adolescents," Gatorade Sports Science Institute Sport Science Exchange #77, accessed January 15, 2015, http://www. gssiweb.org/sports-science-exchange.

213 Bob Davis, interview by Grace Lee, 2014.

214 Caroline Mahoney et al., "Effect of Breakfast Composition on Cognitive Processes in Elementary School Children," *Physiology and Behavior* (2005): 635.

215 "Healthy, Hunger-Free Kids Act," United States Department of Agriculture, last modified March 3, 2014, http:// www.fns.usda.gov/ school-meals/healthy-hunger-free-kids-act.

216 "Smart Snacks in School," United States Department of Agriculture, last modified January 12, 2015, http://www.www.fns.usda.gov / healthierschoolday/tools-schools-smart-snacks.

217 Amber J. Hammons and Barbara H. Fiese, "Is Frequency of Shared Family Meals Related to the Nutritional Health of Children and Adolescents?" *Pediatrics* 127, no. 6 (2011): e1565, doi:10.1542/ peds2010-1440.

218 Nicole Larson et al., "Eating Breakfast and Dinner Together as a Family: Associations with Sociodemographic Characteristics and Implications for Diet Quality and Weight Status," *Journal of the Academy of Nutrition and Dietetics* 113, no. 12 (2013): 1601, doi: 10.1016/j.and2013.08.011.

219 "Calcium—Dietary Supplement Fact Sheet," accessed January 31, 2015, http://www.ods.od.nih.gov/factsheets/calcium-healthprofessional/.

220 Michael B. Zemel, "Role of Calcium and Dairy Products in Energy Partitioning and Weight Management," *American Journal of Clinical Nutrition* 79, no. 5 (2004): 907S–912S.

221 David Schardt, "Milking the Data," Center for Science in the Public Interest, Nutrition Action Newsletter, September 2005.

## CHAPTER 10

222 Chad Kerksick et al., "International Society of Sports Nutrition Position Stand: Nutrient Timing," *Journal of the International Society of Sports Nutrition* 5, no. 17 (2008), doi:10.1186/1550-2783-5-17.

223 Ibid.

224 Ibid.

225 Christine A. Rosenbloom and Ellen Coleman, *Sports Nutrition—A Practice Manual for Professionals*, 5th ed. (Chicago: Diana Faulhaber Publisher, 2013), 5–9.

226 Ibid.

227 Kerksick et al., "Nutrient Timing."

228 Rosenbloom and Coleman, *Sports Nutrition—A Practice Manual for Professionals*, 5th ed., 5–9.

229 Ibid.

230 Ibid.

231 Kerksick et al., "Nutrient Timing."

## CHAPTER 11

232 Doris Jane Lutz, interview by Grace Lee, 2014.

# INDEX

*g* denotes graphic; *t* denotes table

surgery, supplements and, 50
sweat, 57, 180–182, 185–187, 188,
    189, 190, 192, 193, 199,
    210, 215, 217, 219, 250, 253
sweeteners, 17, 203, 204
synbiotics, 33
systemic inflammation, 109

**T**

tannins, 82
tap water, vs. bottled water, 191
taurine, 59, 194, 201
tea, 8, 32, 55, 56, 82, 112, 196,
    198t, 208
teens
    calcium shortfall in, 238–242
    creatine and, 54–55
    heat and hydration in,
        207–212
    nutrition challenges for tennis
        kids, 226–232
    nutrition tips for tennis
        parents and coaches,
        232–237
    supplements and, 50–51
tempeh, 32
Tennissmith, 156
testing for illegal substances, 47
testosterone, 62
thermic effect (of food), 162
thiamin (vitamin B1), 41
thirst, 181
"Tips for Dietary Supplement
    Users: Making Informed
    Decisions and Evaluating
    Information" (FDA), 49
tofu, 13t, 28, 29t, 31, 36, 75t, 82,
    107, 152

Tolerable Upper Intake Level
    (UL), 64
tournament play, 90, 144, 151,
    208, 209, 254
toxins, 87, 111
trace minerals, 42, 130
Tracy (case study), 213–214, 223
trail mixes, 135, 174, 221
trans fats (trans-fatty acids), 100,
    101–103, 112, 113, 114, 118,
    127, 133, 216, 221, 234
triglycerides, 97, 100, 129,
    140, 204
Tsonga, Jo-Wilfried, 84
turmeric, 44
25-hydroxyvitamin D, 26
type 2 diabetes, 14, 15, 129, 228
Tyson, Mike, 78

**U**

ulcerative colitis, 109
ultraviolet (UV) rays, 20
ultraviolet B light (UVB), 25,
    26–27
unhealthy menu/healthy menu
    makeover, 117–118
United States Tennis Association
    (USTA), 232, 258
unsaturated fats, 96, 97, 105,
    114, 115, 249. See also
    monounsaturated fatty acids
    (MUFAs); polyunsaturated
    fats/polyunsaturated fatty
    acids (PUFAs)
US Anti-Doping Agency, 48
US Department of Agriculture
    (USDA), 3, 7, 10, 15, 21,
    37, 243. See also Dietary

# Acknowledgments

I would like to acknowledge and express my deep appreciation to Andrew, Ben and Anthony – my number one fans – for their patience and cheers. To my mother who still instills work ethic, integrity and grit in her classy, dignified way.

To my co-tennis player friends who inspire me with their drive to be better players and better people. Thank you for sharing your story and asking me all those diet questions on and off the court.

To the great tennis legends who graciously offered their wisdom, including Nick Bollettieri, Doris Jane Lutz, Steve Smith, Jimmy Arias and Bob Davis. Bob's volunteerism is beyond admirable. Their accomplishments humble me.

To friends and colleagues who provided professional support and expertise: Ann Clifford McGough, Ray Collins, Bob Davis, Eric Davidson, Mario Carrillo, Susan Hicks, Kathy Whyte, Bill Rompf with *Play Sarasota* magazine, the nutrition experts at Cornell University, and the friendly staff at Total Tennis of Sarasota, Florida.

# About the Author

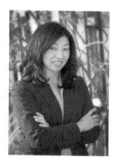

Grace Lee, MS, RDN, earned a bachelor's and master's degree in human nutrition from Cornell University. She has been a registered dietitian/nutritionist for more than twenty-five years and is an avid tennis player. She is contributing writer for *Play Sarasota* magazine and volunteer nutrition educator for the Panda Foundation, addressing childhood obesity through tennis, nutrition, and life lessons. She has two children, Andrew and Ben, and resides in Sarasota, Florida.

Printed in the United States
By Bookmasters